The Ultimate Non-Dairy Keto Diet Guide For Women Over 40

Lose 20 Pounds in 30 Days

T. M. Holcombe

CONTENTS

Introduction

G

etting in shape was as easy as denying yourself that extra scoop of ice cream or committing to a regular exercise program when you were in your teens and early twenties. However, as you get older, you are dealing with all sorts of bodily changes. Weight loss after 40 is notoriously difficult for women in particular due to childbirth; we struggle to get rid of that "child weight." In addition to stubborn fat, we also must deal with a slower metabolism, decrease in muscle mass, increase in calorie intake, hormonal changes, low activity, and the normal stress that comes with life. Nonetheless, getting older doesn't mean you have to accept the fact that you will always need to upgrade your wardrobe every time you need to go up one size. It is definitely possible for women that are older than 40 to lose weight. It does not have to be a constant struggle over the course of your life, but for women over 40, it can be quite challenging.

Now, you might ask why bother writing another weight loss book. The answer is simple. Most of us who are serious about losing weight and keeping it off are doing it all wrong or we are just not committed to it. To be honest, when I was growing up I never had weight issues. I never struggled with my diet. I was very comfortable at 140 pounds. I also had a nice, plump butt, which made me look good in any pair of jeans. I was healthy and I did not overeat. While thinking about it, I must admit that I was very active back then. I played volleyball at IS 51 on Staten Island and I also did a lot of walking. Of course, I was also a regular at the Wyandanch High School gym and I did some gymnastics and basketball there as well. Yes, I moved a couple of times, but I always stayed active. For example, when I moved back to Brooklyn, my sister and I were part of the Eastern District High School basketball team. We had dance in our gym classes along with aerobics. In short, staying active was the reason why I never gained a significant amount of weight.

This remained the case until I had my children and started a desk job that required me to sit for hours. That is when I started to gain a significant amount of weight. By the time I had my last child at the age of forty-two I weighed 224 pounds. My stomach was the main culprit. It was always poking out, making me look like I was pregnant. I absolutely hated it when people asked me if I'm pregnant. I had to get bigger shirts to camouflage my fat stomach. I started to purchase those "squeeze me until I can't breathe" under garments which just ended up hurting me and making me use the bathroom way more often than it was necessary. So, there I was, 224 pounds and the mother of six children. I was definitely taking care of my family, but hardly taking care of myself. I was tired all the time and not eating right. During the ninth month of the pandemic, my tiredness became so overwhelming that I had to see a doctor. I was taking frequent naps and I could not stay awake. My primary doctor sent me straight to the hematologist because according to him my blood count was low. Believe it or not, I had to get iron infusions every week for a month. I could have ended up with multiple other health problems, as well as needing a blood transfusion. I was setting myself up for a life of health issues. In those moments I thought about everything, especially what would happen if something bad happened to me and I was no longer here for my children. Almost every single person in this world wants to live a long life and I am no exception. I would like to be healthy and be there for my children. I want to see them grow and I want to give them advice when needed along with my love and all of my support. However, the reality is that I can't do that if I'm not here. That is the main reason why my attitude and my thoughts about healthy living changed. This was an eye-opener. I need to get healthy to be able to live for me and my children. I started to think about losing weight and getting healthy. I did extensive research and I found that the ketogenic diet was one of the best ways I could maximize my health while losing weight. I also noticed that by eliminating all milk products I would lose even more weight. Since I changed the way I eat and the way I feel about food, I have been happier, lighter, more motivated, and less stressed. I lost 14 pounds after the first three weeks when I tried this method. Within the next month, I lost 21 pounds. One day I asked myself, what else can I do? Well, I can write a book that will help women like me, all over the world improve their lives by giving them a guide into understanding how to get back healthy and in shape. With this book, they will be able to follow my steps into a weight loss journey of their own and lose a significant amount of weight.

You know, it takes consistency and effort to shed pounds at any age, but this is even more so the case for women over 40. My recommendation would be not to try to lose weight quickly after turning 40 because sustainable weight loss always happens more gradually as a result of making healthy lifestyle changes over time. In no time at all, you can be on your way to a stronger and healthier you. Continue reading to learn why people put on weight after they turn 40 and how you can lose that weight and keep it off for good!

CHAPTER ONE

Losing Weight When You're 40 Or Older

E

ven if you've never had a problem maintaining your weight, the gradual creep of extra pounds becomes harder to manage the older you get. This is a fact and it is scientifically proven. So why is this happening? There are a few different factors at play. For one, fat is likely sticking around longer on your body. According to one research done not that long ago, a process called lipid turnover (how quickly your body removes fat) gets slower as you age. The result is body fat that just won't budge as quickly as it used to. Hormones also play a role. Women have a drop in estrogen and men have lower levels of testosterone—two things that can make it harder to lose weight and can lead to more abdominal fat, especially in women. That shift can also cause muscle loss. On average, people lose between three and 8% of their muscle mass every decade after they turn 30. That impacts how many calories your body burns throughout the day. Muscle is more metabolically active than fat, so loss of muscle can lower your metabolism and cause gradual weight gain. Unless physical activity increases or you cut back on the amount of food you're eating, weight gain usually happens.

According to my research, there are seven main reasons why it is extremely hard for women to lose weight. Those reasons are:

Pregnancy

Children can bring a lot of joy to a family; however, many women are sometimes left with the unwanted features of childbirth. They include stretch marks, cut vaginas, abdominal cramps, swollen breasts and feet, dry mouths, and an expanded stomach. With all these added stresses to pregnancy, there is no wonder many women will go through postpartum depression. Before you can lose weight after pregnancy you must focus on healing.

Decrease in Metabolism

Metabolism is the set of life-sustaining chemical reactions in all organisms. The three main purposes of metabolism are converting the energy found in food to energy available to run cellular processes; converting food to building blocks for proteins, lipids, nucleic acids, and some carbohydrates; and eliminating metabolic waste. These enzyme-catalyzed reactions allow organisms to grow and reproduce, maintain their structures, and respond to their environments. The word metabolism can also refer to the sum of all chemical reactions that occur in living organisms, including digestion and the transportation of substances into and between different cells, in which case the above-described set of reactions within the cells is called intermediary (or intermediate) metabolism. In various diseases, such as type 2 diabetes, metabolic syndrome, and cancer, normal metabolism is disrupted (Smith, Reuben, Soeters, Maarten, Wust, Houtkooper, Riekelt, 2018).

Metabolic reactions may be categorized as catabolic (the breaking down of compounds such as glucose to pyruvate by cellular respiration) or anabolic (the building up or synthesis of compounds such as proteins, carbohydrates, lipids, and nucleic acids). Usually, catabolism releases energy, and anabolism consumes energy (Newsholme, Arthur, Start, 1973).

The chemical reactions of metabolism are organized into metabolic pathways, in which one chemical is transformed through a series of steps into another chemical, each step being facilitated by a specific enzyme. Enzymes are crucial to the metabolism because they allow organisms to drive desirable reactions that require energy and will not occur by themselves by coupling them to spontaneous reactions that release energy. Enzymes act as catalysts. They allow a reaction to proceed more rapidly and they also allow the regulation of the rate of a metabolic reaction, for example in response to changes in the cell's environment or to signals from other cells (Smith, Reuben, Soeters, Maarten, Wust, Houtkooper, Riekelt, 2018).

The metabolic system of a particular organism determines which substances it will find nutritious and which it will find poisonous. For example, some prokaryotes use hydrogen sulfide as a nutrient, yet this gas is poisonous to animals. The basal metabolic rate of an organism is the measure of the amount of energy consumed by all of these chemical reactions. Unfortunately, as we get older, our metabolisms slow down. Why?

- **Loss of muscle mass.** As you age, you naturally lose muscle mass. As a result, you burn calories at a lower rate.

- **A less active lifestyle.** As you get older, you may get less physical activity than you used to. Not getting enough exercise can lead to weight gain and cardiovascular disease. These conditions also contribute to the slowing of your metabolism.

- **Gender and genes.** These also play a role in your metabolism rate. Men typically have a faster metabolism because they have more muscle mass, heavier bones, and less body fat. Genes determine your muscle size and ability to grow muscles. These affect your metabolism, too. The less muscle mass you have, the slower your metabolism becomes.

When does our metabolism slow down?

- At 30. By this age, you may notice that losing weight isn't as easy as it used to be. This happens because as you get older, you move less. If you aren't physically active, you could lose 3% to 5% of muscle mass each decade.

- At 40. Your body starts to lose muscle mass naturally. This process is called sarcopenia. Even if you're active, your body will still lose some muscle. During this time, fat will start to form instead of muscle. This also slows down your metabolism, depending on how much muscle mass you've lost.

- Other factors. Hormones and genetics will also impact how quickly your metabolism slows down as you get older. Every person has a different mix of these, so it can be hard to predict the rate at which your metabolism is slowing down.

To be honest, the lower metabolism rate is quite visible if you pay a bit more attention to it. To be more specific, take a piece of cake and eat it. Do you feel like you gained a pound after eating it? Probably, yes. Now, go back in time. I bet that you did not feel like this in your 20s. I bet back then you felt like you could eat an entire cake and never gain an ounce. I think that you have even thought about this before and no, it is not in your imagination. As previously said, as we age, our metabolism slows and the rate at which we break down food decreases by 10% each decade after we turn 20. In short, by the time we are 50, we experience a 30% drop (Smith, Reuben, Soeters, Maarten, Wust, Houtkooper, Riekelt, 2018).

A slowing metabolism can lead to weight gain each year even if you don't eat much more than usual. For example, if you eat a bowl of ice cream every night (amounting to about 500 calories) you will have consumed 3,500 extra calories that week, which amounts to a pound of fat. Multiply this by 52 weeks a year and you can see a significant weight gain from consuming just one extra treat a night (Newsholme, Arthur, Start, 1973).

Maintaining muscle mass is the key to preventing weight gain, but it can be challenging because after they turn 45, the average person loses an estimated 1% of muscle mass each year. The muscle mass is the second reason why women find it hard to lose weight after a certain age.

Less Muscle Mass

From the time you are born to around the time you turn 30, your muscles grow larger and stronger. But at some point in your thirties, you start to lose muscle mass and function. The cause is age-related sarcopenia or sarcopenia with aging. Physically inactive people can lose as much as 3% to 5% of their muscle mass each decade after this age. Even if you are active, you'll still experience some muscle loss.

There's no test or specific level of muscle mass that will be diagnosed as sarcopenia. Any loss of muscle matters because it lessens strength and mobility.

Muscle mass plays a huge role in our health. So much so, that sarcopeniaand sarcopenic obesity (the combination of low muscle mass and excess fat), and dynapenia (the loss of muscle strength) are associated with a surprisingly wide range of health conditions, from heart disease and diabetes to frailty and dementia.

Increased Calorie Intake

Consistently binging on unhealthy or junk food on the weekend could be hurting your weight loss goals. Research suggests that exercise alone may not contribute to substantial weight loss without sufficient changes to the diet. Most people who have difficulty losing weight are simply eating too many calories. An important factor in weight loss is how many calories you're eating versus how many calories you're burning. It may seem easy, but if you're not tracking your calories each day, you may be consuming more than you think (Redman L, Heilbronn L, Martin C, 2007).

Next comes stress. Stress can significantly impact your ability to maintain a healthy weight. It can also prevent you from losing weight. Whether it's the result of high levels of the stress hormone cortisol, unhealthy stress-induced behaviors, or a combination of the two, the link between stress and weight gain is glaring.

Stress

Researchers have long known that rises in cortisol can lead to weight gain. Every time you're stressed, your adrenal glands release adrenaline and cortisol and as a result, glucose (your primary source of energy) is released into your bloodstream. All of this is done to give you the energy you need to escape from a risky situation (also known as the "fight or flight" response). Once the threat has subsided, your adrenaline high wears off and your blood sugar spike drops. This is when cortisol kicks into high gear to replenish your energy supply quickly. Cue the sugar cravings. Because sugar supplies your body with the quick energy it thinks it needs, it's often the first thing you reach for when you're stressed. The downside to consuming so much sugar is that your body tends to store sugar, especially after stressful situations. This energy is stored mainly in the form of abdominal fat, which can be particularly hard to shed. And so the vicious cycle starts: get stressed, release cortisol, gain weight, crave more sugar, eat more sugar, gain more weight.

Here is another twist that you had no idea that I am about to mention. Remember, the first reason? The lower metabolism? Well, lower metabolism happens due to cortisol as well. Namely, even if you aren't eating foods high in fat and sugar, cortisol also slows down your metabolism, making it difficult to lose weight. In 2015, researchers from Ohio State University interviewed women about the stress they had experienced the previous day before feeding them a high-fat, high-calorie meal. After finishing the meal, scientists measured the women's metabolic rates (the rate at which they burned calories and fat) and examined their blood sugar, cholesterol, insulin, and cortisol levels. The researchers found that, on average, women who reported one or more stressors during the prior 24 hours burned 104 fewer calories than non-stressed women. This could result in an 11-pound weight gain in one year. Stressed women also had higher insulin levels, which is a hormone that contributes to fat storage (Ohio State University, 2015).

Increased levels of cortisol can not only make you crave unhealthy food, but excess nervous energy can often cause you to eat more than you normally would. You might find that snacking or reaching for a second helping provides you with some temporary relief from your stress but makes healthy weight management more difficult. When we are stressed and not planning, we tend to eat the first thing we see and/or what is readily available and accessible, which is not always the healthiest options. You may also be more likely to go to a fast-food drive-through, rather than taking the time and mental energy to cook a balanced, healthy meal.

Balanced, healthy meals are easy to cook but somehow, we end up with food that is low in vitamins and minerals. I found out that the lack of vitamin and mineral intake is yet another reason why we can't lose weight. In fact, this lack of intake is causing weight gain in three different ways.

Lack of Vital Minerals and Vitamins

Individuals who get the least nutrients end up weighing the most, and those who get more nutrients end up weighing less. In medical language, individuals with the lowest intake of vitamins and minerals have the highest BMI. Weight gain happens due to:

- **Cravings**: Low nutrient levels in the appetite center of the brain can trigger a ravenous appetite and uncontrollable cravings! Our brain's appetite center has receptors that know if we are deficient in key nutrients, like iron, vitamin D, or B-complex vitamins. If we are deficient, our appetite center gets turned on and we will eat more. Often the cravings are excessive, relentless, and irresistible, especially for tasty, high calorie foods that cause excessive weight gain.

- **Fatigue**: Low nutrient levels cause fatigue, limiting activity. When we are tired, we are less active. Chores, shopping, and fitness activities just don't get done! This fatigue, often the result of missing key nutrients, will sabotage the best intentions to be fit and active. More unwanted weight gain occurs from less activity.

Once again, this is about a slower metabolism. Do you see how everything is actually connected? Missing nutrients slows the metabolism. Essential nutrients play key roles in our body chemistry. Nutrients build muscle and bone, create energy, burn sugar and fat, and keep mood elevated. If you aren't getting all your vitamins and minerals, a slower metabolism will also contribute to progressive, unwanted weight gain.

Hormones and Perimenopause

Weight gain during peri-menopause can be caused by a number of different factors, including hormonal changes, and is commonly felt most keenly around the stomach area. However, it is important to look at the full picture and take a holistic approach when determining the cause of weight gain during menopause, as lifestyle, mental health, and genetic factors could all play a role.

As you get older, your metabolism slows down and your body burns calories at a slower rate. Therefore, if you continue to eat in the same way as you always have, but don't increase the amount of exercise you do, you are likely to experience weight gain during menopause.

Similarly, many people reduce the amount of exercise they do as they get older, which leads to muscle breakdown and more fat.

Unhealthy eating continues to be a big risk factor for gaining weight during menopause, particularly when combined with a slower metabolism.

Looking at your family history can also be an indicator of potential weight issues during menopause, as a genetic predisposition to weight gain at this time is common. As you get older, it is not unusual that maintaining your weight becomes more difficult. Weight gain during menopause and perimenopause is one particularly common issue. It's not an inevitable symptom of menopause, instead, it is one of the most visible ones.

During perimenopause, the first hormone that decreases is usually progesterone. This can lead to estrogen dominance, a common symptom of which is weight gain around your stomach area.

It can often be confusing to hear that estrogen dominance is one of the primary factors that lead to weight gain during menopause, as it is commonly understood that estrogen levels drop during this time. Whilst it is true that your estrogen levels drop significantly during menopause, if your progesterone levels decrease at a faster rate, you can still become estrogen dominant, no matter how little estrogen you actually have in your system. As long as you have lower levels of progesterone than estrogen, you are likely to experience many of the symptoms associated with estrogen dominance.

Low Activity

Inactivity, rather than overeating, could be driving the surge in women's obesity. Examining national health survey results between 1988 and 2010, the researchers found huge increases in both obesity and inactivity.

Energy balance is a process through which the body attempts to establish homeostasis. Most individuals spend much of their lives in the same weight range without daily focus on caloric intake and output. The two parts of the equation for weight maintenance are energy intake (eating and drinking) versus energy output (non-exercise thermogenesis + exercise). To achieve weight loss, most researchers recommend exercise as an integral part of any weight loss program. Physical activity and exercise are often used interchangeably. However, correctly defined, physical activity is all movement that creates energy expenditure, whereas exercise is a planned, structured physical activity. Research supports the importance of exercise in relationship to improved cardiovascular fitness, insulin sensitivity, glycemic control of type 2 diabetes, blood pressure, and depression scores. But does exercise itself contribute to weight loss and maintenance efforts? Indeed, it does. Physical activity of all types, including aerobic exercises, resistance exercises, flexibility exercises, and reduced sedentary time, clearly results in multiple health benefits for individuals with type 2 diabetes and should be included in any lifestyle recommendations for individuals with diabetes. Encouraging women to exercise for longer periods of time each day helps to enhance weight loss. However, it is challenging for some patients to consistently achieve even small bouts of exercise daily as they get older. That is the main reason why we gain weight that easily.

Remember when we all dreamed about working from home? Now, that's a reality for 42% of the U.S. labor force. And while there are some perks to not having to step inside an office (like not having to wear a tie or heels), there are some downsides. Some of them, like weight gain, can take a toll on your health. We spend only about seven hours out of every 24 standing and moving. Our sedentary jobs now cause us to burn 100 fewer calories a day than we did 50 years ago. That alone can translate into an extra 10 pounds of weight gain every year.

Other less known reasons why women in their 40s get overweight or obese

- A lot of women simply continue to eat the same amount of food that they did when they were younger even though they're less active. That makes it easy for them to gain weight without changing anything else (Mozaffarian, Dariush, Hao, Rimm, Walter, Willet, Hu, 2011).

- Hormonal changes that occur as we age contribute to weight management. For example, we develop a resistance to leptin, a protein hormone that regulates energy intake and expenditure. It's also believed that aging plays a role in reduced responsiveness to thyroid hormones. These hormonal changes in senior adults can contribute to an increase in fat mass.

- There are genetic factors that play a role in senior obesity. It's believed that certain genotypes produce a different sensitivity to changes in body fat after overeating (Mozaffarian, Dariush, Hao, Rimm, Walter, Willet, Hu, 2011).

- Believe it or not, our environment contributes to the chances of putting on weight as we age. Some seniors have less access to exercise and fitness centers, especially those who can offer specialized weight and physical activity programs. Seniors need safe places to walk and bike, and these aren't always readily available (Mozaffarian, Dariush, Hao, Rimm, Walter, Willet, Hu, 2011).

CHAPTER TWO

Obesity Factors

I

t is obvious that you are reading this book because you are overweight. Otherwise, you'd be drinking cocktails on the nearest beach, and not stressing over finding possible solutions for your problem. This chapter is focused on the road that took you to this book. I wrote this chapter because I want you to find out exactly what mistakes you made and how you gained weight. After learning about them and remembering them you will become much stronger and more resilient in the future.

You are now forty years old or more. Think about your 20s and your 30s. Yes, they just flew right by. When I think about my 20s and 30s, I can say that I ate a lot of unhealthy things but at the same time, I was quite active. I was always going somewhere, always acting on something. Of course, I also engaged in many unhealthy habits back then. As much as I regret many unhealthy habits, I cannot change the past. Life really comes at us fast. You also probably have families and children you want to care for and be present in their lives. For this to happen, you need to take care of yourself. Obesity kills.

There are dozens of reasons as to why we are here in the same predicament and fighting for our lives. We are fighting because this is a struggle and as much as we want to win, we are not winning this battle. However, your purchase of this book tells a whole different story. It says that you are a fighter and you will never be satisfied with your life unless you get your weight under control. The same applies to your happiness, health, and mental wellbeing. We can't erase the past and the bad habits that we had back then, but we can eliminate those bad habits right now and create newer, better habits. After all, old habits are the ones keeping us heavy, uncomfortable, and filled with low self-esteem. Believe it or not, when we ae not comfortable with specific areas of our lives, we do not perform at our peak. So, regardless of how we arrived in this awful place; let's do something different now to make permanent changes. But before that, let's look at how we ended up here. The two most useful measures for characterizing excessive fat are body mass index (BMI) and waist circumference. BMI is calculated based on a person's weight and height and gives a reasonable estimate of total adiposity. A BMI between 18.5 and 25 kg/m2 is considered acceptable, while a BMI equal to or greater than 30 usually indicates obesity. A waist circumference measurement gives an indication of the amount of fat stored within the abdomen and this distribution of fat has been associated with worse health outcomes. In males, a waist circumference equal or greater than 102 cm is usually considered very high risk, while in females the corresponding value is 88 cm.

The Obesity Factors

Measuring weight may be relatively simple but defining when it has become a health risk is more difficult. Obesity can be defined as a condition of excess body fat where the fat has accumulated to an extent that it is likely to be detrimental to health. However, obese individuals are not all the same; they vary considerably in the degree of excess body fat, the distribution of the fat within the body, and the health risks associated with the excess fat.

Research has long attempted to define the key determinants of obesity and there remains a degree of controversy over which factors have made the greatest contribution to the recent rise in the rates of obesity in the world today. As we established in the first chapter, food intake and physical activity behaviors are the two key factors that have the potential to directly influence energy balance and weight status. Much discussion has revolved around the relative influence of specific behaviors. Key dietary behavior linked to creating energy excesses include a high intake and increasing portion size of energy-dense foods, especially high fat foods; snack foods and food eaten away from home; a low intake of high fiber, low energy-dense foods, especially vegetables and fruit; and a high consumption of sugar-sweetened beverages. Physical activity changes over time are hard to document but it appears that leisure time physical activity has not declined substantially over the last three decades, while there have been substantial reductions in occupational and incidental physical activity. At the same time, the amount of time spent sitting or being sedentary has increased dramatically.

The changing social, political and physical environment in which we live tends to encourage obesity-promoting behaviors and discourage appropriate eating and physical activity behaviours. Urban design and the built environment discourage physical activity and active travel and influence the ease of access to appropriate food. Changes in the food supply have led to the wide availability of cheap, high kilojoule processed foods that are aggressively marketed. The portion size of snack foods, sweetened drinks, and takeaway foods has increased and their relative cost has decreased, while the relative cost of fresh produce has increased. Changes to occupational structures and work environments have led to the replacement of physically active workplaces with desk-bound and sedentary occupations. In addition, longer working hours leave less time for food preparation and family recreation and physical activity. Disrupted sleep patterns exacerbate the lack of time for planned activity and food preparation.

Further, powerful genetic and physiological processes that are geared to the accretion of energy for survival undermine attempts to limit energy intake and increase energy expenditure. In particular, our genes and nutrition exposures in utero and early in life have profound effects on our regulation of energy balance and how and where we store fat generated by excess kilojoules.

There are certain times in a person's life when they are more prone to weight gain and thus require special focus in addressing the problem. Critical life stages for weight gain include the prenatal stage, the time of adiposity rebound (5–7 years), adolescence, early adulthood, pregnancy, and menopause.

The Process of Weight Gain

Weight gain occurs when there is an energy surplus that is sufficiently large and sustained for long periods. It is not well defined how much of an energy surplus is required to initiate weight gain but it is known that the relationship between excess energy and the amount of body energy stored in fat is not linear or direct. When energy intake increases above expenditure, weight gain occurs but does not continue indefinitely. This is partly because as new adipose tissue is created, the energy cost of maintaining that new tissue also increases, thus decreasing the overall energy surplus. Over a period of time, the increases in weight will lead to a situation where the increased energy expenditure has totally eroded the energy surplus and a new equilibrium is created.

Behaviors

Food consumption and physical activity behaviors are the two key factors that have potential to directly influence energy balance and weight status. Historically they have been considered a product of free will under the direct cognitive control of the individual. However, as previous sections have indicated, there is a range of biological as well as social and environmental forces that constrain these behaviors in individuals. However, an appreciation of the dietary and activity behaviours that have been linked to weight gain and the development of obesity is important if we are to usefully define these problems and decide how best to address them. Both energy expenditure and energy intake contribute to weight gain and the development of obesity and it is not possible to clearly apportion the contribution that each makes to the problem. There has been a lot of unnecessary debate over which factor is more important in the genesis of obesity. Attempts to selectively promote one factor over the other as the major cause are counterproductive, as both will need to be addressed in tackling the problem.

Dietary behaviors

A number of dietary factors have been identified as potential contributors to weight gain and obesity by undermining the innate regulatory control of body weight. There are multiple mechanisms by which this can occur, including satiety, palatability, food availability, and low energy needs as a consequence of physical inactivity.

Go to almost any town in the country and you'll find a couple of fast-food restaurants. Is fast food to blame for the obesity epidemic? It plays a huge part. In larger cities, you'll find a string of chain restaurants that are lined up to offer consumers the opportunity to take their pick. The food that is available in these eating establishments is generally not the best thing that you can put in your body. Much of it can be considered junk food. It's usually high in calories and fat. It's processed food that is packed with additives and is often fried before it's slapped on a plate or put in a wrapper. Fast food costs less and it's quick. It's also easy to buy in large quantities and overeat.

In fact, it's easy to put two and two together to link fast food and obesity. Burgers at McDonald's or Burger King contain well over 500 calories and include the entire amount of fat that you should have in a day. Add the fries and you're talking about more than 300 calories added to the meal. If you go for fast food, you're more likely to pick a soda for a drink, which means empty calories with a beverage that is high in sugar. One meal at a fast-food restaurant is probably going to run up to around 1,000 calories. You do the math. If you eat this way on a regular basis, especially if you grab fast food for lunch and dinner, you are headed for disaster.

Bad Habits

When a behavior relating to food intake or activity is repeated often for a long period of time, it becomes a habit, meaning that it becomes almost an automatic response to certain cues or situations. Habits often remain well after the original reason for adoption of the behavior has passed, making them difficult to change. Often, people passively adopt or continue a behavior rather than making an active decision to do so. Once habits are formed, individuals show little inclination to change them. In addition, attitudes and intentions have less of an impact when a habit has been established, making changes to inappropriate food and activity behaviors less likely even when the need for such a change is accepted. Food and activity habits are often associated with an increased energy intake, and as environments become more "obesogenic" (obesity-promoting), the behaviors that lead to obesity are increasingly the default or automatic ones.

Genetics

To date, more than 400 different genes have been implicated in obesity, although only a handful appear to be major players. Genes contribute to the causes of obesity in many ways, by affecting appetite, satiety (the sense of fullness), metabolism, food cravings, body-fat distribution, and the tendency to use eating as a way to cope with stress. The strength of the genetic influence on weight disorders varies quite a bit from person to person. Research suggests that, for some people, genes account for just 25% of the predisposition to be overweight, while for others the genetic influence is as high as 70% to 80%. Having a rough idea of how large of a role genes play in your weight may be helpful in terms of treating your weight problems (Harvard Health Publishing, 2019).

Genes are probably a significant contributor to your obesity if you have most or all of the following features:

- You have been overweight for much of your life (Harvard Health Publishing, 2019).

- One or both of your parents or several other blood relatives are significantly overweight. If both of your parents are obese, your likelihood of developing obesity is as high as 80% (Harvard Health Publishing, 2019).

- You can't lose weight even when you increase your physical activity and stick to a low-calorie diet for many months (Harvard Health Publishing, 2019).

- Genes are probably a lower contributor for you if you have most or all of the following features:

- You are strongly influenced by the availability of food (Harvard Health Publishing, 2019).

- You are moderately overweight but you can lose weight when you follow a reasonable diet and exercise program (Harvard Health Publishing, 2019).

- You regain lost weight during the holiday season, after changing your eating or exercise habits, or at times when you experience psychological or social problems (Harvard Health Publishing, 2019).

Sleep

The correlation between sleep and weight gain occurs for a handful of reasons. When you don't get enough sleep and need more energy, you may find yourself reaching for excess amounts of food to provide the necessary fuel. Research shows that the less sleep you get, the more likely you are to store fat and take in more calories. When you are tired, you tend to reach for food or caffeine to keep you going. Because of this, adequate sleep (at least seven and a half hours) is important to maintain weight levels.

Sleep and Hormones

Lack of sleep also has an impact on your hormones that can promote weight gain and insulin resistance. Sleep deprivation is associated with obesity and diabetes. In fact, studies show that as little as two days of sleep deprivation is enough to result in hormonal changes that promote weight gain and insulin resistance. The hormones that regulate your appetite are greatly influenced by how long you sleep. This means that a lack of shut-eye causes an increase in appetite that may be excessive for your daily needs.

Two major hormones control hunger. ghrelin and leptin. Ghrelin is a hormone that is released when our body is hungry. It stimulates appetite and promotes fat storage. Leptin has the opposite effect. It suppresses the appetite, telling your body you are not hungry. It also encourages the body to burn fat. Studies show that those who are sleep-deprived may have increased ghrelin levels and decreased leptin levels, causing increased food intake, especially foods high in carbohydrates and sugar. This is because of your increase in hunger and decrease in energy. To ensure a lack of sleep isn't affecting your hunger level (and many other important functions of the body), prioritize getting at least seven hours of quality sleep.

Stress

As if stress wasn't pesky enough, many people are unaware that it has a sneaky effect on weight. When our stress levels are high, our cortisol (stress hormone) increases. This decreases insulin sensitivity and can cause weight to be stored around our midsection.

To be clear, this means that those stress cravings aren't purely psychological. The decrease in insulin sensitivity—and, therefore, increase in insulin levels—that happens when you're anxious leads to a drop in blood sugar. This stimulates your appetite.

Moreover, recent studies are looking into how stress affects weight on a molecular level. Glucocorticoids or the body's natural steroid cells are produced when the body is trying to fight inflammation.

The body's level of glucocorticoids naturally rises and falls throughout a 24-hour period. However, if the body is in a constant state of stress during both day and night, glucocorticoid levels are constantly high. As opposed to the usual rise and fall, this causes a higher conversion rate of fat cells than usual. It's important to note that more research on this particular reaction is needed.

Hydration

As if you needed another reason to drink plenty of water, getting too little can impact your weight, as well as tons of important bodily functions. When we don't get enough water to aid our body to work correctly (for example, with digestion, temperature regulation, and lubrication of the eyes and joints), our cells signal the brain that we need more fluid.

Sometimes, people can confuse these thirst signals with hunger signals and eat instead of drinking, causing weight gain. To make sure you're not confusing the two, always check in with yourself and stay hydrated throughout the day.

On the other hand, drinking plenty of water can cause weight loss. Studies also show that increased hydration can aid to increase metabolism and lipolysis, the process of fat breakdown, aiding in weight loss. If you consistently drink a lot of fluids and find yourself having an easier time losing weight, that may be why.

Medications

Medications causing weight gain can be a tricky subject, especially because everyone reacts differently to them. Before we get into it, note that everyone's body is different.

If you've gained an unusual amount of weight since starting a medication, consult with your doctor. Some medications (like antidepressants) can cause carb cravings or water retention and bloating. This typically depends on the individual and their response to the medications. Some medications can also simply make it more difficult to lose weight. So, you have to be even more consistent and careful. Some of these drugs include birth control pills and steroids.

Other possible side effects of medications include a stimulated appetite, a decrease in metabolism, an increased storage of body fat, and an impaired tolerance to exercise. Classes of medications with possible weight change side effects include antihypertensives (e.g., beta blockers such as metoprolol and calcium channel blockers), diabetes medications (e.g., insulin and sulfonylureas such as glyburide, glipizide, and thiazolidinediones), steroids (e.g., prednisone, chemotherapy drugs, and contraceptive pills), antidepressants (MAOIs such as trazodone and SSRIs such as Zoloft and Remeron), antipsychotics for mental illness, and anticonvulsants for neurological conditions such as epilepsy (e.g., gabapentin and pregabalin).

Conversely, certain medications can suppress your appetite, causing unintentional weight loss. These include medications for cancer, HIV, and dementia. If you experience any of these symptoms, do not hesitate to inform your doctor.

The Environment Factor

As I explained above, our genetics are responsible for helping us gain weight and stay overweight. However, the environmental factors are those outside forces that additionally complicate the problem. Namely, they include anything that is present in the environment you live in that makes people more likely to consume a lot of food or to exercise as little as possible. A lot of experts indicate that environmental factors are driving force for the causes of obesity and the rise of it (Harvard Medical School, 2019).

The problem becomes more intriguing after understanding that these environmental influences started contributing to the problem even before you were born. Researchers focused on obesity and environmental issues name these in-utero exposures "fetal programming." This means that every baby that comes from a mother that smoked during pregnancy is more likely to become overweight (Harvard Medical School, 2019). You never thought about this, right? On the other hand, the babies of mothers that did not smoke during their pregnancies ended up not being overweight. The same happens with mothers that have diabetes. Conditions like diabetes alter the baby's metabolism while growing in ways that show up later in life.

I spoke about habits earlier but not about childhood habits precisely. These types of habits sometimes do not leave us, and they remain inside of us even after growing up and entering adulthood. A lot of children that drink sugary sodas and consume processed foods that are high in calories take their need for them into adulthood. As they keep consuming them, they gain enormous amounts of weight. Children that watch television while growing up and play video games all the time remove physical activity from their lives and are programming themselves for a sedentary future.

In short, a lot of modern life promotes obesity. Our environment continuously encourages us to exercise less but eat more. And there's growing evidence that broader aspects of the way we live—such as how much we sleep, our stress levels, and other psychological factors—can affect weight as well.

Regardless of the reasons you're in the predicament you're in, a change must be made. You have to become able to force yourself to change some of your behaviors in order to start promoting weight loss instead of continuing down the same path. Make a personal commitment just as I did.

The Dangers of Being Overweight

While weight-related chronic diseases lead to high rates of mortality in people of all ages, the risk of dying from weight-related disease increases as people age. Additionally, it's proven that older adults who struggle with obesity also have higher rates of depression. The lungs of obese women decrease in size, making it easier to develop respiratory problems. Because as we grow older, we naturally lose about 20% of our skin's dermal thickness, older adults who are overweight and obese can develop pressure sores much more easily. Being overweight or obese as a senior can cause and/or exacerbate serious conditions such as type 2 diabetes, cardiovascular disease, and osteoporosis (Mozaffarian, Dariush, Hao, Rimm, Walter, Willet, Hu, 2011).

In this chapter, we found out that multiple lifestyle changes are independently associated with long-term weight gain, including changes to the consumption of specific foods, physical activity, and metabolism. During my research, I discovered that alcohol use, television watching, and smoking also play a significant role and can lead to weight gain.

CHAPTER THREE

Making A Personal Commitment

A

t the very beginning of this chapter, I want to tell you that you need to understand and determine your "why." Why do you want to lose weight? Why is it important for you to start losing weight? These are the two questions that I continuously asked myself before I started. I answered them differently each time and I understood that "why" is important when you want to lose weight and start taking your health seriously. The consequences of not losing weight should also be familiar to you and I included them at the end of this chapter.

Now, you noticed the name of this chapter. Commitment is a word that we use often. If you check its meaning in the Oxford Dictionary, it means "the state or quality of being dedicated to a cause, activity, etc." People make commitments all the time, that is why this word and the action it represents are commonly used. We commit to staying in school. We make commitments to finish a 200-piece puzzle but when the puzzle gets too hard, we quit. Also, we make commitments to our relationships but quite often we fail to hold them true. There are times when we are not committed to anything at all. A lot of people do not commit to anything and anybody and live a relaxed life. Commitment takes time and trust. Sometimes, it leads to uncomfortable situations. We can learn a lot from these uncomfortable situations as we grow through them and become better. With all of this in mind, I would like to invite you to make the biggest commitment of your life. I invite you to make a commitment to regain control of your weight, your health, and your mental well-being. After all, without commitment, we do not stand a chance of winning this war. So, at this moment I want you to do one thing. Please say these words, "I am fully committed to winning this struggle with my weight. I am committed to changing my lifestyle in order for me to live a longer, healthier, happier, and less stressful life." With that being said, let's continue our journey fully committed and ready.

The beginning of this chapter includes some of the most common myths and facts that surround obesity. There are plenty of misconceptions and myths about it due to the rising rates of this affliction. Yes, there is a lot we do not know about the cause of obesity and the best way to manage it depends on different factors but for sure we do know a lot more than we used to and we know the difference between facts and myths. I think that you should know these things as well before you fully commit. Despite the lack of supporting data, members of the public, mass media, and the government often advocate mistaken beliefs. This only makes the problem worse.

Myth Number One: Obesity Happens Due to Poor Life Choices
Fact Number One: Obesity Is Multifactorial

If you take a look online, you will see that a lot of people blame obesity on poor diet choices and lack of physical activity. A lot of times there are comments that indicate that people with obesity lack motivation or are "lazy."

Yes, as we established before, diet and lack of exercise are important factors when it comes to obesity but there are many other factors that contribute to it. To be even more factual, most people, even those that are not obese, do not complete the recommended amount of physical activity each day.

Myth Number Two: Weight Loss Will Fix All Your Health Issues
Fact Number Two: If Not Done Properly, Weight Loss Can Cause Health Issues

Weight loss involves many systems in the body that are responsible for storing energy. Weight loss can reduce your risk of heart disease, diabetes, and other complications. But the disruption of the body's energy systems can also lead to other health issues. These issues associated with weight loss can make it more difficult to sustain it over time.

Weight loss can improve your overall health but it's also associated with psychological stress, hormone disruption, and metabolic complications. Losing weight too fast can increase your risk of muscle loss and lower your metabolism. It can also cause nutrient deficiencies, sleep issues, gallstones, and other complications. Some people may develop sagging skin and stretch marks as a result of weight loss. Sometimes, weight loss can affect your mental and emotional health as well.

Myth Number Three: Weight Loss Is "Calories In vs. Calories Out"
Fact Number Three: The Above Statement Fails to Understand the Complexity of Weight Loss

I know that you have heard the phrase above. If somehow you didn't, what it means is that if one wants to lose weight, one must burn more calories than one consumes. While the importance of calories for weight loss can't be denied, this type of thinking is far too simplistic. Macronutrients like proteins, fats, and carbohydrates can have diverse effects on your body.

The calories (type and amount) that you consume affect the amount of energy you use. The foods you eat can also affect hormones that regulate when and how much you eat. Some foods can cause hormone changes that encourage weight gain. Another problem with the idea of losing weight based on caloric intake is that it ignores the other health effects of foods. Eating to get the most nutritional benefits is essential for preventing diseases and staying healthy over time.

Myth Number Four: The Lost Pounds Are the Greatest Measure of Success
Fact Number Four: Success Is Measured by Health, Not Pounds

All too often, weight loss and healthy eating programs focus on the numbers on the scale. But focusing on weight loss as the only measure of success is not only ineffective but it's also psychologically damaging.

Focusing only on the scale can lead to cycles of weight loss and gain. It can also lead to heightened stress, disordered eating, self-esteem issues, and an unhealthy obsession with your body image. The key to long-term success is to focus on making healthy choices about your diet and exercise, not on the amount of weight you've lost.

Growing evidence suggests that shifting the focus of success to weight-neutral outcomes, like blood pressure, diet quality, physical activity, self-esteem, and body image is more effective than using weight loss as a measure of success (Jeffery RW, SA, Forster JL, 1991).

Myth Number Five: Making Fruits and Vegetables Accessible Will Solve the Problem of Obesity

Fact Number Five: Lack of Education on the Obesity Topic and Food Preferences Play a Bigger Role than simply Making Fruits and Vegetables Accessible

A lot of people think that the obesity issues can be solved by making vegetables and fruits more affordable and accessible. That applies in locations where obesity is prevalent. Many cities and states have already implemented policies to increase the number of grocery stores and farmer's markets in so-called "food deserts." These are places with limited access to fresh, healthy food. Food deserts are commonly found in low-income areas.

However, education and preferences play a stronger role in making healthy food choices, more so than income and accessibility. Improving people's diets requires making food accessible and affordable on top of regulating the number of unhealthy food options in a community. Plus, it requires changing people's knowledge about diet and health. This approach includes promoting diets rich in fruits and vegetables. It also involves reducing people's consumption of unhealthy foods.

Obesity is serious because it is associated with poorer health outcomes and reduced quality of life. Obesity is also associated with the leading causes of death in the United States and worldwide, including diabetes, heart disease, stroke, and some types of cancer (NHLBI, 2013). In the following part of this chapter, I am going to talk about the health risks of obesity.

Doctors generally agree that the more obese a person is the more likely he or she is to have health problems. People who are 20% or more overweight can gain significant health benefits from losing weight. Many obesity experts believe that people who are less than 20% above their healthy weight should still try to lose weight if they have any of the following risk factors.

Common Health Risks Caused by Obesity
Obesity and Your Mind

Several research studies have found that obesity is linked to mood and anxiety disorders. This means that if you are obese, you may be more likely to suffer from a mental health condition like depression or anxiety (Kissebah, H., Freedman, & Peiris, 1989).

You may be wondering if obesity causes mental health issues or vice versa. The nature of the relationship between obesity and mental health differs from person to person. For some people, emotional distress may lead to overeating. Food can serve as a way to cope with stress, which can result in excessive weight gain and obesity.

For others, obesity may cause emotional distress. Being overweight can lead to negative feelings about oneself. People who are overweight may also encounter judgment or stigma from others. These experiences can lower self-esteem. People who are obese may find it difficult to participate in positive activities, which can make it harder to cope with negative emotions. Additionally, obesity is linked to having more physical health problems and pain, which can increase stress (Kissebah, H., Freedman, & Peiris, 1989).

Diabetes

Women who are obese have a high risk of developing type 2 diabetes, which is also known as insulin-resistant diabetes or adult-onset diabetes. This is a condition in which your blood glucose level is persistently high. Research suggests that people who are obese are up to 80 times more likely to develop type 2 diabetes than those who are not. In obese persons, cells of fat tissues have to process more nutrients than they can manage. The stress in these cells triggers an inflammation that releases a protein known as a cytokine. Cytokines then block the signals of insulin receptors, thus gradually causing the cells to become resistant to insulin. Insulin allows your cells to use glucose (sugar) for energy. When you are resistant to insulin, your body is unable to convert the glucose into energy and you end up with a persistently high blood glucose level. Besides suppressing normal responses to insulin, the stress also triggers inflammation in cells that can lead to heart disease (Kissebah, H., Freedman, & Peiris, 1989).

Cardiovascular Disease and Stroke

Heart disease and stroke are the leading causes of death and disability for people in the U.S. Overweight people are more likely to have high blood pressure, which is a major risk factor for heart disease and stroke, than people who are not overweight. Very high blood levels of cholesterol can also lead to heart disease and are often linked to being overweight. Being overweight also contributes to angina (chest pain caused by decreased oxygen to the heart) and sudden death from heart disease or stroke without any signs or symptoms.

The frequency of heart failure in obese people is increasing; it is one of the major causes of death globally with a prevalence of approximately 3% in developed countries (Kissebah, H., Freedman, & Peiris, 1989). A close correlation can be observed between heart failure and obesity. According to data from the Framingham Heart Study, the rise of BMI by 1 kg/m2 increases the risk of heart failure by 5% in men and 7% in women (Kissebah, H., Freedman, & Peiris, 1989). Studies on heart failure show that 32%–49% of patients suffering from heart failure are obese and 31%–40% are overweight. In the case of obese and overweight patients, heart failure develops 10 years earlier than in the case of subjects with a normal BMI. The duration of morbid obesity is closely correlated to the development of heart failure. After 20 years of obesity, the prevalence of heart failure grows by 70% and after 30 years, the prevalence rises by 90% (Kissebah, H., Freedman, & Peiris, 1989). The significance of obesity is indicated by the fact that the Framingham Heart Study emphasized the pathogenic role of obesity for the development of heart failure in 11% of males and 14% of females (Kissebah, H., Freedman, & Peiris, 1989). The structural and functional changes of the heart observed in obesity alone contribute to a deterioration in myocardial function, which is often referred to as "obesity cardiomyopathy" (Kissebah, H., Freedman, & Peiris, 1989).

Obesity leads to heart failure through several direct and indirect mechanisms. Excess weight leads to haemodynamic changes. A rise in both cardiac output and blood pressure has been observed; an increase in BMI of 5 kg/m2 involved a 5 mmHg rise in systolic blood pressure (Kissebah, H., Freedman, & Peiris, 1989). On one hand, it is related to the activation of the renin-angiotensin-aldosterone system and on the other hand, to the increased activity of the sympathetic nervous system (Kissebah, H., Freedman, & Peiris, 1989).

Medical scientists have found that being overweight leads to high blood pressure, which is one of the leading causes of stroke. Being overweight also leads to metabolic syndrome□—characterized by high cholesterol, high triglycerides, and high blood sugar. Over time, these conditions harm the blood vessels of the brain and the heart and increase the risk that a blood clot will form and travel to the brain☐, resulting in a stroke. When researchers compared people with metabolic syndrome to non-sufferers, they found that people with metabolic syndrome are three times more likely to have a stroke.

Cancer

The link between obesity and cancer risk is clear. Research shows that excess body fat increases your risk for several cancers, including colorectal cancer, post-menopausal breast cancer, uterine cancer, esophageal cancer, kidney cancer, and pancreatic cancer. What's less clear is exactly how being obese increases this risk. Experts believe that it's largely due to the inflammation caused by visceral fat, which is the fat that surrounds your vital organs (Kissebah, H., Freedman, & Peiris, 1989).

The problem with excessive visceral fat is that it affects certain processes in your body. This includes how your body manages hormones like insulin and estrogen. All of this can lead to an increased cancer risk by affecting how and when cells divide and die.

Visceral fat cells are large and there are a lot of them. This excess fat doesn't have much room for oxygen. Low-oxygen environments trigger inflammation. Inflammation is the body's natural response to injury and disease. For example, when you get a deep cut, the areaaround the cut becomes red and painful to touch. This minor inflammation around the wounded area helps repair the damaged tissue and aids with the healing process. But long-term inflammation caused by excess visceral fat can damage your body and increase your risk of developing cancer. Cancer happens when cells reproduce uncontrollably, damaging the cells around them and causing illness. The more cells divide and reproduce, the higher the risk that something will go wrong and a tumor will form (Kissebah, H., Freedman, & Peiris, 1989).

The link between inflammation and insulin (the hormone that regulates blood sugar) is complex. Inflammation caused by obesity can keep the body from properly responding to insulin. This is called insulin resistance. When the body doesn't respond to insulin correctly, it produces more insulin to make up for that. The increase in insulin due to insulin resistance triggers an increase in the number of cells produced, which can lead to cancer. Increased insulin also affects how hormones like estrogen are controlled. More insulin can lead to more available estrogen, which increases cancer risk (Kissebah, H., Freedman, & Peiris, 1989).

Basically, higher estrogen levels lead to increased cell production, which could result in tumor growth. Estrogen is necessary for the body to function. In women, the ovaries are the main source of estrogen. In men, an enzyme converts testosterone to estrogen. But fat cells in both men and women can also make estrogen. This is high levels of estrogen are commonly seen in obese people. In women, too much estrogen is linked to an increased risk for post-menopausal breast, endometrial, and ovarian cancers (Kissebah, H., Freedman, & Peiris, 1989).

Liver Disease

People with obesity can develop liver disease known as fatty liver disease or nonalcoholic steatohepatitis (NASH). This happens when excess fat builds up in the liver. The excess fat can damage the liver or cause scar tissue to grow, known as cirrhosis. Fatty liver disease usually has no symptoms, but it can eventually lead to liver failure.

Gallbladder Disease

The gallbladder is responsible for storing a substance known as bile and passing it to the small intestine during digestion. Bile helps you digest fats.

Obesity increases your risk of developing gallstones. Gallstones occur when bile builds up and hardens in the gallbladder. People with obesity may have higher levels of cholesterol in their bile, or have large gallbladders that don't work well, which can lead to gallstones. Gallstones can be painful and require surgery.

Pregnancy Complications

Pregnant women who are overweight or have obesity are more likely to develop insulin resistance, high blood sugar, and high blood pressure. This can increase the risk of complications during pregnancy and delivery, including:

- Gestational diabetes
- Preeclampsia
- Needing a cesarean delivery (C-section)
- Blood clots

- Heavier bleeding than normal after delivery
- Premature birth
- Miscarriage
- Stillbirth
- Defects of the brain and spinal cord in the fetus

In one study, over 60% of women with a BMI of 40 or greater when they got pregnant ended up having one of these complications (Kissebah, H., Freedman, & Peiris, 1989).

Believe it or not, but obesity is linked with reproduction as well. Namely, it can influence a lot of aspects of reproduction. Among women, the association between obesity and infertility, primarily ovulatory infertility, is represented by a classic U-shaped curve. In the Nurses' Health Study, infertility was lowest in women with BMIs between 20 and 24 and increased with lower and higher BMIs. This study suggests that 25% of ovulatory infertility in the United States may be attributable to obesity (Harvard Medical Review, 2020).

Osteoarthritis

Osteoarthritis is a common joint condition that most often affects the knee, hip, and lower back joints. Carrying extra pounds places extra pressure on these joints and wears away the cartilage (tissue that cushions the joints) that normally protects them.

Besides all of the above health risks that obesity causes, there are a couple of more reasons why you need to finally commit to your weight loss journey.

Often, regardless of how funny it sounds, people compare body fat with ATMs. Yes, they think it is a place where we deposit energy or withdraw it from. Well, it isn't. Body fat is an active endocrine organ. That means that it secretes hormones and cytokines (cell signaling molecules). Hormones and cytokines have effects throughout the body. They "talk" to one another chemically. Like all things, balance is important. If we have a healthy amount of fat, our hormones and cell signals work properly. If we have too much, things go wrong. For example, with too much body fat, our immune systems get off-kilter. There's a huge, scary pile of evidence here so let's keep it simple. Increased BMI and high levels of body fat are associated with greater risk for several kinds of infections including gum infections, nose and sinus infections, stomach infections, and herpes. Why?

Too much adipose (fat) tissue can release large amounts of immune chemicals. Over time, this chronic high exposure can interfere with the body's ability to spot and stop actual outside infections. So, losing body fat can translate into a healthier, more responsive, and more robust immune system. And that means fewer colds, fewer infections, and a healthier daily life.

A good night's sleep is another reason. More body fat means more potential for sleep apnea. This comes from a few combined factors:

- Fat in airways narrows the space available for breathing. This makes your airways more prone to collapsing.

- Fat in your upper body puts weight on your lungs and reduces the space available to them. You need more oxygen, but you can't get it as well.

- Fat—a hormone-producing organ—changes your hormonal

signals. This rewires your respiratory systems.

Sleep is a major regulator of our metabolism. If our sleep is bad, so is our metabolic health. This means that things like elevated inflammation, rapid cell aging and oxidation, and hormonal disruption (and, yes, higher risk for all kinds of nasty chronic diseases in the long term) all happen when we don't sleep well. So, lose weight is so that you can sleep better. Not only does this help regulate metabolism, hormone systems, and more. It also helps you feel, think, and live better right away.

The third and last reason is the taste of your food. This reason is not familiar to people and after reading it, you will feel a bit confused. Don't. It is known that people who struggle with their weight don't taste food as people who do. Obese people have altered taste perceptions leading to eating more and eating more of the wrong foods. By losing weight you'll end up craving less high-sugar food. You might even enjoy an extra veggie or two.

How to Finally Commit?

Have you ever watched a motivational speaker? His delivery is on fire! And everyone is so pumped they could literally burst out of the venue and get to work. Their motivation is off the charts! Two weeks later... Check back on them and you'll find 99% of them are right back where they started. They haven't made any progress and their motivation is nowhere to be found. And what's the very first thing someone says? Well, that they were not committed. To be honest, I agree. But, let's turn commitment into something solid, something real, and most importantly – something that we can control!

Usually, when we say we don't feel committed to losing weight, what we really mean is:

We don't feel like doing this anymore. It's too damn hard! And just to be clear, it's not a problem of IF we want to lose weight. I wanted to lose weight for years. That's not the problem at all. The real reasons are that:

- We've lost focus on the reason why we started.

- We've come to the realization that what we're doing isn't sustainable.

And when those two things happen, I can guarantee you that you'll want to quit. Once we know why we don't feel committed, we can fix it.

- First thing to do: Focus on the WHY. Write down why losing weight is important to you and read it today, tomorrow, and the day after that.

- Second thing to do: Make your plan sustainable. Be confident enough that you can perform each action required for successful weight loss.

Mental Strategies That Have Helped Me Lose Weight

How do we keep ourselves motivated to continue to put in the work? It's hard to do! If it was easy, "lose weight" wouldn't have a permanent spot on our New Year's resolution. I offer two mental strategies up two tactics that will continually stoke the fire:

1. **Use weekly check-ins to celebrate small successes**. Recognizing your wins keeps you motivated. Check in with yourself every Sunday about your progress for the week and specifically what went well. When you did a good job, you should recognize that because it keeps you motivated. Then you can go back and reflect. It'll remind you of your progress and of the things that you did really well; you need that. Part of the sustenance of keeping with a goal is feeling good about yourself. Take five minutes each Sunday to complete this journaling prompt: What did I do well this week? What didn't go well this week? What can I do differently next week to improve?

2. **Plan ahead and find your intrinsic motivation to do it.** It sounds simple, but there's truth to the adage: "Those who fail to plan, plan to fail." For busy people, planning ahead is the

most efficient way to get done what you need to get done— whether it's your job, your workout, or meal planning. It's not easy and we have so many things going on. Putting things down on paper clears your brain. Now you don't have everything in your head; it frees up the space to focus on what you need to do. Set time aside on Sunday to plan out the week ahead. Planning is important from an organizational perspective. When it comes to organizing, you really need to think about what's important to you. I always tell people, don't over-schedule. You don't have to say yes to every single invitation. Think about what your week is going to look like and how you're going to find time for what's important.

CHAPTER FOUR

The Non-Dairy Keto Diet

T

here is a saying that it takes 10,000 hours to master a skill. Assuming this is true, I am most definitely a master of dieting. For the better part of two decades, I've spent a pretty embarrassing amount of time worrying about my weight, my pants' size, the amount of food I ate, the amount of food I didn't eat, and how many calories I could burn in a given day.

As you already know, I have tried everything and once I figured out what works best for me I wrote this book. Besides the plan that I included in the 4th chapter, the keto diet plan is the second thing that worked for me and helped me lose weight.

Like so many others, I found out about ketogenic diets online. In fact, I found out about keto while browsing weight loss progress pictures one night. Having just stopped eating a high-carb, raw vegan diet because of how terrible it made me feel, my interest in a better way to eat was definitely piqued.

I saw so many dramatic before-and-after photos, all touting keto as the secret to those results. After spending the night reading through the keto subreddit, I decided to give it a shot. After all, I had just discovered that high carb wasn't the way to go for me. Why not try the opposite approach?

I went all in. I noticed results pretty quickly. I dropped 5 pounds after the first week. After three months, I had lost the 20 pounds that were plaguing me, all without making any other changes to my lifestyle.

Aside from the weight loss, I noticed other improvements in my well-being. My digestion had normalized for the first time in my life. While going gluten-free earlier in the year had certainly helped ease my symptoms of irritable bowel syndrome (IBS), keto brought about a dramatic change in how my digestive system functioned. Without going into too many details, let me just say that I finally understood what doctors and fiber supplement ads mean when they talk about being "regular."

In addition to the digestive changes, I experienced a decrease in joint pain and swelling symptoms I didn't even realize I had until they weren't there anymore. I woke up feeling well rested, found that I could think more clearly, and even had more energy throughout the day.

The Keto Diet: What Is It?

In a nutshell, a ketogenic diet is a high-fat, low-carbohydrate, moderate-protein way of eating that shifts your body from burning glucose (sugar) for energy to a state of ketosis, in which your body preferentially uses ketone bodies and fat as a fuel source. Your liver creates ketone bodies from fat when your body needs to make energy but no glucose is present. This process most commonly occurs during periods of carbohydrate restriction, very limited food intake, and intense exercise. Acetoacetate and beta-hydroxybutyrate are ketone bodies; acetone (a by-product of their breakdown) is often considered a ketone body as well (Freeman, Kossoff, Hartman, 2007).

Most people in the world right now are burning glucose as their primary source of energy. When you eat something with carbohydrates in it, your body breaks down those carbs into simple sugars, the majority of which represents glucose. This glucose is absorbed into your bloodstream, where it triggers the release of insulin by your pancreas. Insulin then calls for the uptake of glucose by your muscles to store that glucose for use as glycogen. Insulin also signals your body to store excess glucose and triglycerides as body fat and halts any fat burning currently going on (Freeman, Kossoff, Hartman, 2007).

Fructose, the sugar commonly found in fruits, agave nectar, and—somewhat infamously—high-fructose corn syrup (among other foods), is processed by the liver, where it is either converted to glucose and sent to the bloodstream (where the above process takes place) or stored as fat (triglycerides) in the liver. Though a very small amount of fructose is converted to triglycerides, over time, consuming excessive amounts of fructose can lead to non-alcoholic fatty liver disease (Freeman, Kossoff, Hartman, 2007).

While some people can go their entire lives burning glucose for fuel without issue, others have problems relying on glucose for energy. For starters, because the body can store only so much glycogen, you need to replenish those stores by eating often. You know that hangry feeling you get sometimes (read: all the time)?

That's a by-product of your blood sugar crashing in the absence of sugar. Mood swings and mood disorders are a surprisingly common side effect of blood sugar dysregulation, and if you are anything like me, you are already well aware of this fact (as is any person who has ever lived with you) (Freeman, Kossoff, Hartman, 2007).

If you've heard of insulin resistance, then you are already aware of another potential issue with burning glucose as your primary source of energy. Over time, overconsumption of carbohydrates can cause your tissues to become less sensitive to the insulin that your pancreas releases. Because the same amount of insulin is no longer achieving the desired effect, your poor pancreas starts to produce more insulin, which just perpetuates this cycle.

In the presence of insulin resistance, circulating glucose levels can remain high, damaging tissues, keeping the body in a state of fat storage, and preventing the body from burning fat that has already been stored. Eventually, insulin resistance can lead to type 2 diabetes, other metabolic issues, and even cardiovascular disease.

On the flip side of this equation, when there is too little circulating glucose in your bloodstream, the release of another hormone called glucagon is triggered. Glucagon tells your liver to convert that stored glycogen back to glucose for use as fuel. Glucagon also tells your body to break down stored fat into free fatty acids for use as fuel. Burning free fatty acids produces ketone bodies, which your brain and body can then use for energy. This is the beginning of nutritional ketosis. If you continue to restrict carbohydrates, your body will continue burning fat as its main fuel source.

Now, something cool about ketone metabolism is that it cuts insulin out of the picture. Instead of fluctuating, insulin and blood sugar levels remain relatively stable. This stability curbs fat storage, reduces food cravings, and promotes the breakdown of body fat (Freeman, Kossoff, Hartman, 2007).

This ease of fat loss and regulation of hunger signals is one of the main reasons so many people (myself included) find themselves sticking with ketogenic and low-carb diets.

Now that you know what a ketogenic diet is, let's talk about how to get started! Like anything else, you can make keto as simple or as complicated as you want. Not everyone is comfortable with weighing out and writing down every bit of food that goes into their mouth, and by the same token, not everyone feels confident in making food choices without having some guidelines to follow.

Fortunately, you can tailor your approach by using one of the two main styles of keto dieting: tracking and lazy keto. You can use either method or switch between them as you like. I often combine the two—taking a lazy keto approach to which foods I choose to eat and then retroactively tracking them because I love analyzing information.

This has definitely changed over time. When I first started keto, I kept track of only net carbs to make things as easy as possible for myself. A few weeks in, I began to track other macronutrients as well. After five or six months, I stopped tracking and embraced a lazy keto approach, and then, as I started blogging more frequently and creating meal plans, I got serious about my tracking game and started looking at both macronutrients and micronutrients.

There is no need to tie yourself toone method over the other. Try out both approaches to see which works better for you!

Tracking

If you're a person who loves data, do I have good news for you! Being a way of eating that focuses on macronutrients, keto lends itself well to aggressive food tracking.

Within the realm of tracking, you can choose to focus on certain aspects (for example, macronutrient ratios or net carb goals) or go all out and track literally everything. There is noone right way to track what you eat.

Tracking Carbohydrate Intake

This is certainly the easiest approach to tracking what you eat on keto. I started out this way, and I find it to be the most user-friendly approach overall. Basically, you focus on tracking your net carbohydrate intake with the goal of keeping it under a certain limit.

In the beginning, I set 20 grams of net carbs as my goal. I kept a running tally of the carbs I consumed throughout the day without stressing about total calories, grams of protein, or percentage of fat. I did this for the first full week until I had become accustomed to this new way of eating; only then did I start to track other targets, like calories, protein, and fat. Having just one thing to worry about really helped me focus and kept keto from becoming toooverwhelming.

Was I eating a super balanced diet? Probably not, but balance was something I ironed out later. I definitely recommend this style of tracking for those who want to have some sort of goal but aren't super excited about having to worry about balancing macronutrients.

You don't need to download an app for tracking your carb intake (although you can use one; see below for a list of apps); a simple notebook will do the trick.

Tracking Macronutrient Percentages

If you're ready for something a little more advanced than keeping track of net carbs, you could consider tracking your intake of total carbohydrates, protein, and fat. For this approach, I definitely recommend downloading an app like MyFitnessPal, LoseIt, or Cronometer. These apps let you set custom macronutrient goals and then give you a breakdown of how many grams of each macronutrient you should eat. Keep in mind that many apps don't have a "net carbs" setting (though Cronometer does!), so you may have to calculate that number manually.

Many people who follow a ketogenic diet like to keep their fat, protein, and carbohydrate intakes within certain ranges:

- Fat intake is typically between 60% and 80% of total calories.
- Protein intake is generally between 15% and 30% of total calories.
- Net carbohydrates are limited to 5% to 10% of total calories.

As you can see, you have a fairly broad range to work within these parameters.

Those on a whole-food vegan keto diet may find themselves consuming closer to 10% of their daily calories in carbohydrates, as nearly all sources of vegan protein also contain carbs.

You can either log your meals preemptively based on what you plan to eat that day or after each meal. I don't recommend waiting until the end of the day to log everything in one fell swoop, as it can be hard to remember every little thing you ate or drank

It might seem a little tedious at first to have to enter everything into an app (or a physical food diary, if your style is more analogue), but after a while, it becomes second nature, and writing everything down usually takes less than two minutes.

Most apps also allow you to track your body weight and measurements so you can see your progress over time.

Ketone Testing

When I first started keto, I wanted to know if I was in ketosis all the time. I'd wake up in the morning and use a ketone test strip. I'd test again when I got home from work. I'd test at night before going to bed, just to see if anything had changed. I was so excited about keto that I wanted to quantify every second of it.

For those first few weeks, it sure was fun, but eventually, the novelty of seeing that little strip turn dark pink wore off, and I began to rely on other signs to see what was going on in my body.

While I do recommend testing at the beginning, it's not necessary to test your ketone levels all the time. If you are seeing results and feeling great, then there's really no reason to go to the extent of doing it all the time. However, testing can be a nice way to figure out your carb tolerance and your protein tolerance and to even see if certain foods kick you out of ketosis.

It's important to remember that over time, as your body becomes more efficient, it will down-regulate the production of ketones. So, while you may still be in ketosis, you may not continue to put up the same high numbers that you did in the beginning. This is totally normal and shouldn't be discouraging!

Whether you are in a light state of ketosis (producing between 0.5 and 1.5 mmol/L of ketones) or a heavier state, you are still in ketosis.

I've said it before and I'll say it again: there is noone "right" way to eat a ketogenic diet. As long as you are in ketosis, you are eating keto. However, there are some guidelines that can help make the ketogenic diet more nutrient-dense and a little easier to follow, especially during the initial adjustment period.

The History of Keto

As we all know, epilepsy is one of the common neurological disorders. It affects 50 million people all over the world and it is diagnosed when a person experiences sudden, recurrent, and unprovoked seizures. They manifest when cortical neurons fire excessively, hypersynchronously, or both, leading to temporary disruption of normal brain function. This might affect, for example, the muscles, the senses, consciousness, or a combination of all these. A seizure can be focal (confined to a specific part of the brain) or generalised (spread widely throughout the brain and leading to a loss of consciousness). Epilepsy can occur for a variety of reasons; some forms have been classified into epileptic syndromes, most of which begin in childhood. Epilepsy is considered refractory (not yielding to treatment) when two or three anticonvulsant drugs have failed to control it.

Why does this matter? Well, this is how the history of keto begins. The keto diet is a mainstream dietary therapy that was created to reproduce the success and remove the limitations of the non-mainstream use of fasting to treat epilepsy. Due to this reason, the keto diet was highly popular in the 1920s and 1930s. However, due to the development of anticonvulsant drugs, it was abandoned. It is not a secret that a lot of people with this issue are able to control it through medication. But there are cases that are highly dependable on the keto diet because drugs do not help them at all. The failure of these drugs is the reason why the keto diet became so successful once again.

But let's go a bit more back in history. As we already established, if you fast or intermittently fast (don't eat anything for a period of time), your body will start to produce ketone bodies from stored fat to make up for the lack of sugar/carbohydrate energy. Well, our ancestors recognized the metabolic health benefits of fasting as early as about 500 BC, unwittingly instigating a state of ketosis (when you limit carbohydrate intake and your body uses ketones as its primary fuel source) and leveraging it for a variety of conditions. Here are just a few known historical instances of fasting used as a medical treatment:

- Ancient Greek doctors used fasting to treat diseases.

- Hippocrates recorded fasting as the only treatment for epilepsy and managing epileptic seizures/seizure control.

- Benjamin Franklin said, "The best of all medicines is resting and fasting."

- Mark Twain wrote, "A little starvation can really do more for the average sick man than can the best medicines and the best doctors. I do not mean a restricted diet; I mean total abstention from food for one or two days."

- In 1914, fasting was used for treating type 1 and type 2 diabetes.

- In 1922, an osteopath named Hugh Conklin had children with epilepsy fast for up to 25 days, providing only limited liquids.

In the early 1920s, a doctor named Russell Wilder from The Wilder Clinic recognized the dangers of fasting for children and explored different diets to see if something else might elicit a similar response as fasting. He discovered that you could mimic the effects of fasting by avoiding sugar and eating a higher fat, low-carb diet. He tested this diet on children with epilepsy (with a very positive outcome) and his diet became the main pediatric epilepsy treatment for many years. Wilder's discovery was the birth of the ketogenic diet.

In the 1930s, new anti-convulsion seizure drugs were developed. Patients and doctors found taking medication easier than making diet changes, so these new drugs became the primary treatment of epilepsy.

It wasn't until the 1970s, when consumers expressed interest in weight loss and dieting, that the ketogenic diet was reborn. But its comeback wasn't immediate. The following timeline showcases the slow but steady growth in keto popularity and uses:

- 1972: A cardiologist named Dr. Atkins published the book *Dr. Atkins' Diet Revolution* expounding his years of medical research on low-carb dieting for weight loss and heart health. This put the higher fat/low-carb way of eating on the map (History of The Ketogenic Diet, 2008).

- 1977: Dr. Phinney, a physician and scientist who spent his life studying nutrition, authored *The Last Chance Diet*—a book promoting a fat and protein drink diet that he developed. However, this drink he created lacked necessary minerals and people became sick, some even dying (History of The Ketogenic Diet, 2008).

- 1988: Dr. Phinney creates The Optifast Diet—a nutritional program centered around fat and protein drink products he created, but with minerals in it. Oprah endorsed it and keto research picked up (History of The Ketogenic Diet, 2008).

- 1990: U.S. television network NBC aired a show about the positive outcome of the ketogenic diet on a two-year-old boy suffering from severe seizures. The show instigated a big spike in PubMed publications relating to keto (History of The Ketogenic Diet, 2008).

- 1992: An update of Dr. Atkins 1972 book was published. Called *Dr. Atkins New Diet Revolution*, it inspired other doctors to publish dieting books based on similar low-carb principles and marked the beginning of the "low-carb craze."

- 1996: The story of the boy from NBC's 1990 TV special was made into a movie starring actress Meryl Streep and sparking a renewed scientific interest in the ketogenic diet.

- The early 2000s: The Atkins Diet was rediscovered and the low-carb movement gained momentum.

- 2013: A study published in a science magazine showed the anti-aging and health benefits of a ketogenic diet. This created curiosity about the keto diet in the paleo and biohacking communities.

- 2015: Famous podcaster Tim Ferriss interviewed Dr. D'Agostino, a keto research scientist, on "Fasting, Ketosis, and the End of Cancer," pushing the ketogenic diet to the top of Google diet searches, where it has remained ever since (History of The Ketogenic Diet, 2008).

There's been an explosion in the keto low-carbohydrate diet over the past several years, both for personal use and in scientific inquiry. The six-year Google search term trend has climbed steadily and continues to climb. Why is keto so much more than a fad diet? Because the health benefits are mounting far beyond its seizure-free antiepileptic beginnings.

Weight loss

One major reason many people switch to keto is the weight loss benefit. In the absence of starchy carbs which convert to blood sugar (glucose), your body burns fat as fuel (both dietary fat and body fat). Fat as your primary energy source keeps you stable and satiated throughout the day and craving less food. Consequently, it's become a popular diet for battling everything from being overweight to being obese. If you plan your meals and eat within your daily recommended macros, you also burn excess fat and help yourself lose weight fast.

Brain Health

The brain loves ketones. Outside of epilepsy, a keto diet improves the outcomes of other neurological disorders and conditions, such as Alzheimer's disease and Parkinson's disease. Keto also helps with concentration, memory, focus, cognition, and decreased brain fog.

Cancer

Researchers are studying keto as an adjunctive dietary treatment for cancer. So far, results are promising. In recent research, keto significantly increased survival time and slowed tumor growth. The tumor types that were included were pancreatic, prostate, gastric, colon, brain, neuroblastoma, and lung cancers.

Although originally used as a treatment for seizures and exploring neurology, our predecessors knew the health benefits of a ketogenic diet. Today, keto research is growing and we are continuously uncovering new, positive side effects and ways in which the keto diet can benefit health and well-being.

There are plenty of different keto diet versions. I used the non-dairy version and it highly benefited me. There are a variety of reasons people remove dairy from their diet, including allergies, intolerance, inflammation, issues with digesting dairy, autoimmune conditions, and skin conditions. Some people, such as myself, remove dairy from their keto diet simply because they are struggling to lose weight while continuing to eat dairy.

Protein Regulation

Dairy contains a significant amount of protein. As you can see below, some cheeses are actually very high in protein. On a keto diet, protein intake should be moderate and eating too much of it can kick you out of ketosis. So, some people avoid dairy to better regulate their protein intake.

Surprise Intolerances

Some people on a keto diet experience a significant glucose spike or ketone decline when they consume dairy, even if they've never been known to have issues with dairy. For anyone on the keto diet for weight loss, this may be enough reason to delete dairy from the diet.

If you've decided you want to be dairy-free and keto, you're probably wondering what you can eat. So many keto recipes contain dairy. Fortunately, there are plenty of options and workarounds.

Plant-Based Substitutions

There are a lot of wonderful dairy-like, keto-friendly products on the market these days. Go to a well-stocked grocer and you may find cashew cream cheese to replace dairy cream cheese or almond yogurt, which is a good alternative to dairy yogurt.

Additionally, often the dairy in recipes can be replaced with non-dairy alternatives. Almond milk or coconut milk can often replace dairy milk in smoothies and baking. Just remember to watch macros when substituting ingredients in recipes and consider investing in a few great dairy-free keto cookbooks.

Prioritize Whole Foods

I'm a huge fan of seeking out whole foods over their processed counterparts. When I talk about processing, I don't mean fermenting, blending, spiral-slicing, or otherwise changing a food in a way that you could change it in your kitchen. I'm talking about food products that are produced in a lab.

I seek out as many whole foods as possible because they tend to be more nutrient-dense and also more difficult toovereat (at least in my experience). While you can obtain vitamins and minerals from supplements, evidence suggests that the sum of the nutritional value of whole foods is greater than their constituent parts. There are so many flavonoids and other beneficial phytochemicals in vegetables, fruits, nuts, seeds, and legumes that appear to work synergistically, with studies demonstrating that therapeutic use of isolated versions of those compounds is often either less effective or wholly ineffective.

Additionally, though protein bars and other packaged snacks are tasty and convenient, you might hurt your chances of entering ketosis if you indulge in these types of treats toooften. Many contain sweeteners that can kick you out of ketosis if consumed in excess. Plenty of dieters have noted that some of the so-called low-carb sweeteners in these bars actually do impact blood sugar in certain people. So, while a bar might claim to have just 3 grams of net carbs, that might not be the case in reality.

Which Foods Are Forbidden on Keto?

I mentioned this before, but I think it is a really important point to address: there are no "forbidden" foods on keto. A ketogenic diet is comprised of any foods that fuel your body and keep you in a state of ketosis. For most people, this means avoiding starches and grains, as well as soda and sugar-sweetened foods, because they are so high in carbohydrates that they are difficult to consume them without being kicked out of ketosis.

Many people also choose not to consume beans or fruit, which are higher in carbohydrates. However, this does not mean that beans and fruit are not "allowed." As long as you eat these foods in small enough quantities that you stay in ketosis, then they are perfectly suitable for a ketogenic diet. I know many keto dieters who budget their daily carbohydrate intake to include hummus because it's just so tasty that it's worth including.

Eliminate or avoid all of the following:

- **Hydrogenated oils**: These oils contain trans fats and are sometimes found in vegan dairy substitutes and nut butters.

- **Sucralose, aspartame, saccharin, and other artificial sweeteners**: Some people notice that artificial sweeteners can cause weight loss to stall and even kick them out of ketosis.

- **Maltitol**: This sugar alcohol causes a lot of gastrointestinal distress and spikes blood sugar to boot.

- **Added sugars**: While most plant-based foods (even spinach) contain some natural sugars, added sugars are easy to avoid. Check nutrition labels for the "added sugars" line and watch out for ingredients ending in "ose." While some people have no problem eating small amounts of added sugars on a ketogenic diet, others find that even a few grams of sugar can kick them out of ketosis. Honey, maple syrup, and agave nectar should also be avoided.

My Top Keto Ingredients

Avocados

Mentioning avocados almost seems cliché because they're so emblematic of both vegan and ketogenic diets. However, there's a reason for that. Avocados are loaded with vitamins and minerals, including significant amounts of potassium and the elusive vitamin B5. They're also absolutely delicious, especially when sprinkled with hemp seeds and nutritional yeast.

Spinach

Yes, frozen spinach. Spinach is a great source of vitamins A, C, and K, as well as manganese, iron, folate, potassium, and calcium. Frozen spinach is awesome because it's cost-effective, ready to go at a moment's notice with zero prep work, and super nutrient-dense. I keep a few bags of spinach (as well as broccoli and cauliflower) in my freezer so that I can add more vegetables to smoothies and dinners with minimal effort.

Nutritional Yeast

Nutritional yeast imparts a "cheesy" flavor to foods. Just 2 tablespoons (10 grams) contains 8 grams of protein and a whole host of B vitamins, all for just 1 gram of net carbohydrates (although the carb counts may differ among brands!).

I tend to add nutritional yeast to creamy sauces and sprinkle it on top of roasted veggies, sliced avocados, and anything masquerading as spaghetti.

Sauerkraut

I love fermented foods, especially lacto-fermented foods like sauerkraut. Not only is sauerkraut rich in sulfur compounds from the cabbage, but the process of fermentation effectively consumes the carbohydrates present in the cabbage.

Fermented foods have demonstrated a whole host of health benefits in studies, from improved digestion and a reduction in inflammation to improved mental health and moods. Emerging research also suggests that certain strains of lactic bacteria even produce B vitamins as a by-product of the fermentation process.

The Dangers of Dairy

Growing up, I have always been told that milk is good for strong bones. I could remember at one point in my life there were so many milk commercials on TV you would have thought milk was the cure-all for all ailments. After I completely eliminated all milk-based products from my diet, I began to feel better. Milk and cheese used to make me so gassy and bloated. Even when I was just using it in my morning coffee, I had stomach problems. Cow's milk is high in saturated fats, which are perfectly suitable for calves. Dairy products can be detrimental to humans in the long run.

Researchers have found that milk is not the cure-all after all. As a matter of fact, milk can be linked to many diseases. Milk is filled with hormones, pesticides, and other toxins that are harmful to humans. Many studies suggest drinking milk can elevate breast and ovarian cancers. More than 10% of Americans are allergic to cow's milk and more than 30% of the people in the world are lactose intolerant.

There are many issues related to dairy consumption. For example, Americans consume an enormous amount of dairy. The intake of the average American is estimated to be over 600 pounds of dairy products per year (Dengfeng, Ning, Wang, Li, Meng, Liu, 2013).

Dairy foods (including cow's milk) have not been part of the diet of adults for the vast majority of human evolution. We've only been consuming these foods for about 7,500 years, (Dengfeng, Ning, Wang, Li, Meng, Liu, 2013) compared to the roughly 200,000 years humans have been around (with our basic biochemical functionality evolving during a few million years before that).

Intensive and successful marketing by the dairy industry have reinforced a broadly ingrained belief that dairy is good for our health. But is it, really? Dairy has come under fire and scrutiny from nutritional experts, scientists, and physicians for its associations with a number of serious health issues.

Dairy is a significant source of female hormone exposure (Dengfeng, Ning, Wang, Li, Meng, Liu, 2013). Commercial cow's milk contains large amounts of estrogen and progesterone, which is a serious concern. This is further exacerbated by modern dairy cows being genetically altered to continuously produce milk, even throughout their repeated pregnancies (Dengfeng, Ning, Wang, Li, Meng, Liu, 2013).

Even milk products labeled "organic" or "no hormones added" usually contain high levels of these problematic hormones, which are naturally produced by cows (even if those cows have not been given any additional hormones for the purpose of the product label).

In both adults and children, milk consumption has resulted in markedly increased levels of estradiol and progesterone in blood and urine, (Dengfeng, Ning, Wang, Li, Meng, Liu, 2013) and dairy consumption in general has been associated with increased levels of circulating estradiol (Dengfeng, Ning, Wang, Li, Meng, Liu, 2013).

Data show that men who drink milk will absorb the estrogens in the milk, which has been found to result in significantly decreased testosterone production/levels (Dengfeng, Ning, Wang, Li, Meng, Liu, 2013).

Pediatricians have expressed concern regarding childhood exposure to the exogenous estrogens in commercial milk because studies showing that early sexual maturation in prepubescent children can be caused by the "ordinary intake of cow milk."

A broad array of multi-centered, peer-reviewed studies has shown that dairy consumption is one of the most concerning and consistent risk factors for hormone-dependent malignant diseases, including ovarian, uterine, breast, testicular, and prostate cancers (Dengfeng, Ning, Wang, Li, Meng, Liu, 2013).

Also, while there is a culturally popular idea that soy foods may cause feminizing effects. Several studies have found that isoflavones (the plant-derived compounds in soybeans with estrogenic activity) do not exert feminizing effects on men, even at high consumption levels (Dengfeng, Ning, Wang, Li, Meng, Liu, 2013). Other studies have found that soy food consumption can be protective against breast cancer. I think we should be far more concerned about the high levels of real female sex hormones found in dairy, the consumption of which results in measurably higher circulating levels of these problematic hormones.

Also, let's speak about casein for a moment, since it is such a big issue that no one ever mentions. Casein, for those that do not know, is the main protein in dairy products. Studies have shown that it facilitates the growth and development of cancer. In fact, some studies even found that cancer development could be influenced more by controlling casein levels in your diet than by exposure to the underlying carcinogen (Dengfeng, Ning, Wang, Li, Meng, Liu, 2013).

Insulin-like growth factor-1 (or IGF-1), a hormone that promotes cell growth and division in both normal and cancer cells, is thought to be one of the mechanisms responsible for this association. IGF-1 appears to be nutritionally regulated and animal protein consumption (including casein from dairy foods) leads to higher circulating levels of this cancer-promoting hormone. For this reason, consuming casein from dairy is associated with increased risk of cancer development and proliferation.

I do not know if you are aware of the following statement but our immune system normally protects us from microbes and other harmful substances. When it loses its ability to recognize and distinguish harmful substances from normal tissues and cells, it can instead mount attacks against our own bodies.

These "self-attacks" can be triggered by exposure to foreign peptides (including animal protein fragments found in dairy) that have similarities to components in the human body. This can result in our immune system becoming "confused" and misidentifying tissues in our body as "foreign" and thus in need of being attacked and destroyed.

Dairy is associated with increased risk of several immune-related disorders (from allergic conditions to autoimmune diseases), many being life-changing and difficult to treat. The associations with type 1 diabetes and multiple sclerosis are particularly concerning.

- **Type 1 Diabetes**. In type 1 diabetes (also called juvenile diabetes or insulin-dependent diabetes mellitus (IDDM)), the immune system attacks the pancreas, resulting in the body no longer being able to produce insulin to regulate glucose. Multiple large-scale studies have identified an association between cow's milk consumption and increased prevalence of type 1 diabetes (Dengfeng, Ning, Wang, Li, Meng, Liu, 2013). One such study found that cow's milk may contain a triggering factor for the development of IDDM," (Dengfeng, Ning, Wang, Li, Meng, Liu, 2013) and another found that "early cow's milk exposure may be an important determinant of subsequent type 1 diabetes and may increase the risk by approximately 1.5 times."

- **Multiple Sclerosis**. In multiple sclerosis (MS), the immune system attacks the insulating sheath of our own nervous system, resulting in a variety of difficult-to-treat and unpredictable neurologic problems. As with type 1 diabetes, numerous studies have reported that cow's milk consumption may be a significant risk factor for developing MS.

Do not get your hopes up about pasteurized milk because it is not good for you either. Milk and other dairy products are important vehicles for foodborne pathogens due to a variety of microorganisms they harbor. Even with modern sanitation requirements, including pasteurization and curing, outbreaks still occur, resulting in severe and sometimes even fatal outcomes.

Salmonella, Listeria, and E. coli are some of the more common foodborne outbreaks associated with dairy. Just last year, for example, three people died from Listeria infections linked to Blue Bell Ice Cream (prompting a large-scale recall by Blue Bell Creameries).

Not even our food regulatory agencies expect milk will be sterile after pasteurization; the heating process is done merely to reduce (not eliminate) the number of microorganisms.

Exposure to organochlorine pesticides (OCP) is another problem associated with dairy. While pesticide contamination affects water and agricultural lands generally, dairy products have a greater capacity to accumulate these pesticides in higher concentrations, due in part to their high fat content (Dengfeng, Ning, Wang, Li, Meng, Liu, 2013).

Even pesticides that have long been banned still show up when dairy products are tested. Some OCPs (like DDT, which was widely used in the past and now banned as a human carcinogen) still persist in the environment and can more easily accumulate in animal food products, including dairy.

In India, milk and other dairy products (like cheese and butter) have been reported as the major sources of dietary DDT and hexachlorocyclohexane (HCH) and routine monitoring detected that milk from dairy farms in Italy's Sacco River Valley had levels of ß-HCH twenty times higher than the legal limit.

Another fact that you are not aware of is the connection between antibiotics and livestock. The largest use of antibiotics worldwide is for livestock. Much of that use is for non-therapeutic purposes, such as infection prevention and to promote feed efficiency and animal growth.

Apart from the dire warnings from scientists that agricultural overuse is leading to antibiotic resistance, another problem is that antibiotic residues persist in milk and other dairy products despite protocols aimed to minimize this.

It is difficult to prevent and control these antibiotic residues because milk from individual cows and farms is usually pooled together and the administration, handling, and record-keeping of animal drug use can vary significantly from one dairy operation to another.

The resulting low-dose antibiotic exposure can lead to a variety of problems, from developing antibiotic resistance to allergic reactions to experiencing side-effects of the medication to which a person is exposed.

Forget about the dairy commercials once and for all. This may come as a surprise to many, but dairy does not appear to be good for bone health, either. Not only has the body of scientific evidence been found inadequate to support the idea that dairy consumption promotes bone health, but numerous large-scale studies have found that consuming dairy may actually be detrimental to bone health. In fact, there are substantial data linking higher milk intake with significantly increased risk of bone fractures.

There are several mechanisms thought to be responsible for the pathophysiology. One is dairy's high calcium content, which can cause vitamin D dysregulation and therefore disrupt bone homeostasis. Another is that the high animal protein content of dairy can induce acidosis from its high proportion of sulfur-containing amino acids, which in turn leads to the body compensating by leaching calcium from the bones to help neutralize the increased acidity. Over time, all of this can have a detrimental effect on bone health.

While several other factors, such as physical activity, can affect bone health, it's significant to note that the U.S. has one of the highest rates of hip fractures in the world, despite our high milk intake. By contrast, in countries like Japan and Peru, where average daily calcium intake is as low as 300 milligrams per day (less than a third of the U.S. daily recommendation for adults), the incidence of bone fractures is actually quite low.

Fortunately, calcium is abundant in plant foods, including leafy green vegetables, legumes and seeds, often with higher absorption rates than the calcium in dairy—and of course without all of dairy's associated health problems.

Each mammalian species produces milk for its own babies, and the content of proteins, fats, carbohydrates and minerals is specific to provide optimum nutrition for a baby of that particular species. The milk from an elephant, tiger, sea lion, and cow is different from one another and they are all different from human milk.

When we think about it, the health problems associated with consuming the milk and dairy products of other species should not come as any surprise. No other species consumes milk regularly past the weaning period and certainly not from another species—and, as mentioned above, humans have also not been doing so for the vast majority of their own evolutionary history (Dengfeng, Ning, Wang, Li, Meng, Liu, 2013).

CHAPTER FIVE

The Importance Of Supplements While Dieting

O

ur bodies work best when vitamin and mineral deficiencies are absent, and healthy food is the best way to get enough of these important nutrients.

The statement above is probably the most important one in this whole book. You should never forget it and you should always try to do as it says. However, the most effective strategy for losing weight is to eat less and move more. Do that and you'll start seeing the pounds peel off consistently. As you do this, however, you lose an enormous number of vitamins and minerals and that is why you should consider adding a multivitamin/mineral supplement to your diet to ensure that you're covered. This is especially important if you happen to have any nutritional gaps, particularly in any vitamin or mineral that may contribute to metabolism.

Before I dive into supplements, I want to stress how important it is to be eating the right foods. Otherwise, taking supplements will be counterproductive. I encourage everyone to do their blood work and to check their vitamin/mineral levels as well. Now, let's talk about supplements. Below is everything that I supplement my program with, as well as some additional suggestions. This is what has worked for me throughout my fitness and weight loss journey. The helpful tips below were given to me by many people, fitness coaches, and nutritionists that I have met during my journey.

Vitamin D

Low levels of vitamin D have been linked to a host of health concerns and conditions, including obesity. You may be low in this super-important vitamin and not even know it. I supplement my diet with vitamin D daily, every morning. Getting enough vitamin D can keep your hormone levels in check and may help enhance weight loss and decrease body fat. In turn, losing weight can increase vitamin D levels and help you maximize its other benefits, such as maintaining strong bones and protecting against illness. We get vitamin D naturally from exposure to the sun, but the winter months prove it to be difficult to get even a fraction of what our bodies need. Some foods have higher levels of vitamin D but consuming enough of those foods may be difficult to reach a therapeutic level. A 2018 study found that overweight women who took vitamin D supplements for six weeks lost more weight than women who did not receive supplements during the course of the study (Maughan, King, Trevor, 2004).

Vitamin C

Vitamin C can assist with weight loss. Whether you want to lose weight or improve strength, vitamin C can help. Being deficient in vitamin C can make it very difficult to lose weight and reach a healthy BMI. It actually helps you to metabolize fat, which is why it is recommended by fitness experts. Vitamin C helps reduce both the physical and psychological effects of stress on our bodies especially while dieting and training. Stress can elevate levels of cortisol and blood pressure and taking a high dose of vitamin C decreases cortisol production. As a woman, you should take 2000 mg-3000 mg per day (Maughan, King, Trevor, 2004). I rarely get sick and I equate that to my vitamin C intake.

Fish Oils

It is recommended that you get a minimum of 2000 mg of fish oil twice daily. The Omega-3 fatty acids in fish oil have various health benefits, one of which is aiding in weight loss. The Omega-3 can help in losing inches as well as body fat, essentially reducing your body fat percentage over time. The Omega-3 fatty acids can also slow down and even inhibit muscle breakdown (which can happen during weight loss) and aid greatly in helping with brain function, liver function, as well as reducing inflammation and lowering triglyceride levels (Maughan, King, Trevor, 2004).

Iodine

For those with an underactive thyroid gland, weight management can be challenging. Iodine is needed to produce thyroid hormones. If you don't get enough, your body can't make enough thyroid hormones and your thyroid, the butterfly-shaped gland in your neck, can't do its job, namely to control your metabolism and numerous other crucial body processes. If someone has a severe iodine deficiency, filling that hole will be valuable for their general health and possibly for weight management.

However, almost no one is deficient in iodine anymore because this mineral was added to table salt in the 1920s. Too much iodine can cause problems including thyroid gland inflammation and thyroid cancer. Talk to your doctor to find out where you stand (Maughan, King, Trevor, 2004).

Iron

Iron is found in your red blood cells or hemoglobin and these cells transport oxygen to the rest of your body. If you don't have enough iron or red blood cells, you aren't funneling oxygen to where it is needed, and this may cause fatigue and other symptoms that make it harder for you to be physically active. But if you don't have a documented iron deficiency, don't take iron supplements. Too much iron is risky and can damage your organs. If you are low in iron, your doctor may suggest eating more iron-rich foods or taking a multivitamin. Have a check-up and also remember that, as a woman, you should include 18 mg daily.

Fiber

Many dieters experience hunger and an increase in appetite and that can lead them to overeat. Fiber makes you feel fuller faster, which leads to weight loss. The average American eats about 15 to 17 grams of fiber per day; the recommended dietary allowance for women is 25 grams. Supplementing your diet with fiber can help you eat less, quell hunger, and lose weight. Increase the fiber in your diet by eating more vegetables. Take an additional supplement if necessary (Maughan, King, Trevor, 2004).

Calcium

Going dairy-free does not mean you must be deprived of your daily calcium intake. There are tons of vegetables that can boost your calcium levels. Examples include collard greens, spinach, turnips, kale, broccoli, and a host of others. This mineral is indispensable to your well-being. It helps maintain bone health but also supports muscle and nerve communication. It helps the cardiovascular system and supports the release of beneficial hormones.

Magnesium

Call it the mighty mineral. As the second most abundant element in the human body, magnesium helps regulate over 300 biochemical functions, including fat breakdown, muscle contractions and cardiovascular health. And yet, roughly 80% of the American population doesn't get enough of this essential nutrient. They—and you—should. Magnesium organically encourages suppler, more radiant skin, hormone balance, bone health, and high energy levels. What's more, healthy magnesium levels may promote deeper, more restorative sleep and sufficient, sound slumber is crucial to weight loss—and to maintaining motivation for a lifestyle change like a new diet.

Probiotics

Probiotics (good quality ones) rebalance the healthy bacteria in the gut. Some research suggests that this can help people to lose weight and belly fat.

Water

Drinking plenty of water is mandatory when dieting, as well as while taking vitamins or fitness supplements. Make sure you are drinking a minimum of eight-ten 8oz glasses of water each day. Staying hydrated while working out is critical. I personally drink one gallon of water every day.

These are the most important supplements that you must include while dieting. Do some experimenting and always discuss any new supplements with your doctor. Get tested to find out your vitamin and mineral levels and make a plan. Consider the foods you eat and decide what to supplement. Both food and pills work and can aid your mental and physical health. Do not forget, they also help you lose weight faster while keeping healthy.

CHAPTER SIX
Additional Weight Loss Boosters

I

f losing weight was easy, there wouldn't be so many diets and approaches to choose from. Every diet and weight-loss strategy has its pros and cons, but for any to really work, you've got to get your mindset right. Now that I've covered many issues about foods, we can discuss how to further improve this understanding into your daily life. Topics such as snacks, shopping, sun exposure, technology, diet, meditation, positive thinking, food preparation, and other eating and drinking issues will be included in this chapter. When it comes to losing weight and getting healthy, we tend to focus primarily on our habits and behaviors, i.e., what we eat and how we exercise, for example. But losing weight is also about our thoughts and beliefs. In other words, it's as much a mental game as it is a physical one.

Snacking

Thus far we've discussed what to eat and how to balance it but there's yet another component to healthy eating habits that can make a positive difference in your health—how often you eat. Specifically, eating more frequently, or snacking between major meals, can improve your health in many ways. In fact, perhaps no other single dietary habit can make a more positive difference in your health than healthy snacking.

In our society, snacks are generally seen as an unhealthful addition of unwanted calories and fat and something to avoid. This can be quite true if you snack on junk food such as candy bars, cake, chips, and crackers that are full of sugar, refined carbohydrates, and unhealthy fats. But healthy, real-food snacks have many health benefits and can help provide you with a continuous supply of the fuel necessary for optimal human performance. Research clearly shows that healthy snacking can help you control blood-sugar levels, improve metabolism, reduce stress and cholesterol, burn more body fat, and increase energy levels.

A healthy snack is just a small meal. The key to healthful snacking is to reduce the amount of food eaten at regular meals and distribute this nutritional wealth throughout the day. Eat five or six smaller meals that add up to the same amount of food that you would normally consume in a typical two- or three-meal-a-day routine. The ideal plan is to start the day with a good balanced breakfast that includes an adequate serving of quality protein. For example, a vegetable egg omelet, a bowl of plain yogurt, and fruit or a healthy smoothie can get your day off to a good start. Skipping breakfast may be one of the worst nutritional bad habits unless combined with intermittent fasting. From breakfast on, plan to eat every two to four hours, based on how it makes you feel. Individuals under more stress or with blood sugar problems usually need to eat more frequently—especially initially, when eating every two hours can quickly make significant changes in overall health.

An example of a daily meal schedule starts with breakfast, a midmorning snack, lunch, a mid-afternoon snack, a light dinner, and if necessary a small snack (which can be a healthy dessert) later in the evening.

Healthy snacks can be almost anything you like, just as long as they are made from real, healthy food. For many people, snacks, like regular meals, should contain protein. Experiment to discover how much food you need and which types work best. Some people may need to eat much larger snacks but others can get by on minimal amounts like just a small handful of raw almonds. This might include:

- Vegetables and fruits such as apples or pieces of cucumber and celery.

- Raw almonds or cashews or almond butter with apple slices.

- Leftovers.

- Non-dairy yogurt and fresh berries.

- A boiled egg.

- Homemade energy bars or healthy smoothies.

The benefits of healthy snacking are various. They quickly suppress cravings, especially for junk foods, they improve physical and mental energy, and they can even stimulate fat-burning by changing your metabolism. Since snacking stabilizes blood sugar and prompts your body to produce less insulin, your body will store less fat and use more of it to fuel all your daily activities from work to play. Many people find that they have much more energy when following a program of healthy snacking.

Snacking can also help your body counteract the harmful effects of daily stress. In this way you reduce the over-production of cortisol and insulin. Both prompt your body to store more fat.

Snacking also helps to reduce cholesterol. Studies show that eating more frequently can lower blood cholesterol, specifically LDL, the "bad" cholesterol. In addition, studies show a staggering 30% increase in heart disease in those eating three meals or less per day.

While snacking has received a bad rap over the years, experts now agree that it was the type of food not the frequency of eating that caused problems. In addition, just piling on the calories by adding snacks to an already unhealthy diet is clearly dangerous. Now we know that eating healthy, balanced snacks throughout the day can help you improve your health in many ways.

Cook Healthy Foods

How and if you cook your food can be just as important as how you select it since even the healthiest ingredients can be reduced in quality through improper kitchen practices. The biggest problems are overcooking, using too much heat, and overheating certain types of oils. There are some guidelines that can help make your work in the kitchen become a work of health. The worst method for cooking anything is deep-fat or high-heat frying, especially using vegetable oils. While many healthy foods may be lightly sautéed in butter or olive oil, deep-frying overheats the oil and can be dangerous. In addition, the high heat may destroy other nutrients in the food itself.

Vegetables can be steamed, stir-fried in olive oil, roasted, baked or grilled. Cook vegetables minimally to avoid destroying vitamins and phytonutrients—they also taste better when not overcooked. If boiling or steaming, use as little water as possible to avoid leaching nutrients.

Eggs can be soft, hardboiled, cooked sunny-side up, overeasy, poached, or lightly scrambled. Use low heat to avoid "tough" or rubbery eggs.

If using oils for cooking it's important to remember that all oils contain varying ratios of monounsaturated, saturated, and polyunsaturated fats. Monounsaturated and saturated fats are not sensitive to heat, but polyunsaturated oils are very prone to oxidizing when exposed to heat. This oxidation produces free radicals, which are related to many health problems. Butter is one of the safest oils for cooking, as it contains a low amount of polyunsaturated fat. Olive oil can also be used for cooking but its polyunsaturated content is a little higher. Another fat you may consider for cooking is coconut oil. In addition, try lard, which contrary to popular belief may be a healthier choice for cooking than butter.

Wine, Alcohol, and Your Health

Wine is not only the oldest alcoholic beverage but the oldest medicinal agent in continuous use throughout human history. The use of wine dates back more than 6,000 years, and is attributed to physicians, scientists, poets, and peasants. Even today, wine and other alcoholic beverages are classified as foods and used daily in most cultures. More healthful benefits have been bestowed upon wine than any other natural substance. For instance, drinking wine with meals can help with relaxation and digestion (German, L. Walzem, 2000).

There are few known unhealthy effects of moderate amounts of alcohol consumption, with negative consequences seen mostly in those who go beyond moderation. Drinking wine and other alcohol in moderation significantly lowers the risk of coronary heart disease. Moderate drinkers have healthier cholesterol ratios because alcohol raises the HDL and lowers LDL. This may be one reason for the lower incidence of heart disease in consumers versus abstainers. Another may be that alcohol increases blood flow to the heart. In addition, alcohol reduces the tendency to form blood clots, a major cause of heart attacks (and strokes).

Alcohol also lowers the risk of Alzheimer's disease and other types of dementiaand improves bone health. Some scientists say that people who have one or two drinks per day may add three to four years of life to their lifespan as compared to those who don't drink.

Scientists also say that red wine may be a potent cancer inhibitor (German, L. Walzem,

2000). Resveratrol, a substance found in red wine (due to the fact that grape skins are used to make red wine), grapes, and thousands of medicinal plants from South Americaand China, not only interferes with the development of cancer, but it may also cause precancerous cells to reverse to normal. Resveratrol also has anti-inflammatory properties.

Most wines contain about 12% alcohol (mostly ethanol, with only a very small percentage of other types of alcohol). Sweet dessert wines may contain up to 20% alcohol. This compares to 40% (80 proof) and 50% (100 proof) alcohol in distilled products such as vodkaand gin. Wine also contains vitamins B1, B2, B6 and niacin, as well as traces of most minerals, including iron. Most red table wine contains iron in its easily usable ferrous form. The pH of wine is low, like that of the human stomach; perhaps this is one reason that wine improves appetite and digestion.

Once in the bloodstream, alcohol is broken down in the liver. About 3.5 ounces of pure alcohol can be safely metabolized by the body if spread out over the day. This translates to about a bottle of wine—not something I'm recommending. To a European, this may not seem like excess, but to an American it might. In the United States, the average annual per-capita consumption of wine is just a few teaspoons, while in Italy, it's about a half bottle.

As a group, women are more susceptible to negative effects of alcohol because of their smaller size, and because they have less amount of alcohol dehydrogenase in their stomachs and livers. This enzyme breaks down much of the alcohol before it's absorbed and in the blood.

If you enjoy wine and want the health benefits associated with it, drink only what you enjoy and can tolerate and no more than one or two glasses. The simplest recommendation is a 4-ounce glass or two with meals. For most people, a glass of wine will be completely metabolized in about an hour and a half. Some people, however, should never consume alcohol.

An obvious side effect of alcohol is that it impairs your senses, so it should be avoided within four hours of driving a vehicle. One drink increases the risk of an accident by 50%, and two drinks by 100%. Also, wine should not be consumed with other drugs or by pregnant women.

Although drinking wine can relax you, any alcohol can disturb sleep if consumed shortly before bedtime. Studies of biological circadian rhythms in humans show that alcohol is best metabolized between 5 and 6 p.m. If you enjoy wine, be sure to ask your doctor whether it poses any health problems for you.

Sunshine

We should love the sun because we can't stay healthy without it. Humans have lived in sunny environments since the beginning of the human race. The sun offers a free source of vitamin D and is the primary source of this important nutrient that has important effects in the body. Vitamin D allows us to more effectively use calcium, improves the immune system, and helps prevents cancer and other diseases.

Based on recent scientific studies, currently recommended vitamin D levels are inadequate, even with the recent increase in recommendations. The average daily need for vitamin D is about 4,000 IUs, but the current recommendation is still only in the 400 IU range from birth to age 50. Recent studies show that more than half the population has inadequate levels of vitamin D—and some of these studies were done in the sunny states of Floridaand Arizona!

In addition to calcium regulation and prevention of cancer, vitamin D specifically helps reduce pain caused by various types of muscle and bone problems. The sun also plays an important role in immunity, especially in children. And the sun is good for the brain—getting natural sunlight helps the brain work better. Obviously, I'm not telling you to stare at the sun! However, allow your eyes to be exposed to natural outdoor light. Contact lenses, eyeglasses, sunglasses, and even windows block the helpful sun rays.

Meditation

When it comes to eating and managing our weight and our health, it is important to acknowledge the importance of the mind-body connection. Our hectic, jam-packed lives may literally be weighing us down.

Specific practices and techniques—meditation, mindful eating, and intuitive eating—can help us learn or relearn how to have a healthy relationship with food and how to remove any problematic feelings we may have about eating. Weight loss may be a side effect of cultivating this renewed relationship, but it's important not to establish losing weight as the primary goal. Doing so may constrain us so that we are unable to truly eat intuitively or in a mindful way (Deikman, 1963).

Instead, focus on enjoying foods—eating because you're hungry, not because you're stressed about work or family issues and feeling overwhelmed. You will learn through these practices how to appreciate and love your body for all it can do for you.

When it comes to talking about meditation for weight loss or meditation for eating and working toward developing a healthy relationship with food, understanding what the terminology means is important.

Stress or emotional eating occurs when people tend to eat or overeat because of strong emotions or feelings, rather than by responding to their own internal cues of hunger. Sometimes when we experience strong emotions, these emotions can outweigh our physical feelings of fullness and satiation and this can result in overeating. In these cases, food is used as a coping mechanism, dulling strong emotions momentarily. However, it's essential to acknowledge that this experience perpetuates a cycle. Feeling stressful emotions can lead to overeating, which leads to guilt or shame, which results in feeling—and not being able to process or handle—negative emotions or stress.

Just as meditation can help us with stress, sleep, focus, and much more, it can also have an impact on our relationship with eating and managing our weight.

Meditation can help us become more mindful eaters and even address any emotional eating issues that might persist. These are described below.

- **Remove the shame and guilt.** For those who struggle with emotional eating, feeling stressed can lead to overeating to soothe themselves or avoid these feelings. This can lead to guilt or shame. Break the cycle. Meditation not only helps reduce stress, which removes the trigger in the first place, but it also helps you become more aware of your emotions and feelings, so you can recognize those times when you're eating when stressed versus when you're actually hungry. Meditation has also been shown to increase our compassion, which may cause us to become more accepting of other people who may have different body types from our own.

- **Maintain weight loss and a healthy weight for the long haul.** Meditation can help your weight-loss efforts stick. While diet and exercise may help you reach your weight loss goals, meditation, alongside healthy eating and exercise, makes weight loss efforts sustainable.

- **Lower stress and inflammation levels.** Meditation reduces cortisol and C-reactive protein levels, which is beneficial to our overall health and may help us achieve weight loss and maintain a healthy weight. Elevated C-reactive protein levels can be a sign of inflammation, which is at the root of many diseases, including obesity.

- **Take better control of cravings.** If you struggle with emotional or binge eating, it can be tough to fight those intense food cravings. Research shows that mindfulness meditation can help us control emotional and binge eating.

- **Decrease stress and anxiety.** Losing weight takes a lot of effort and keeping the weight off can be stressful, even leading to feelings of anxiety. Meditation eases these feelings.

Technology as an Aid

Although some types of technology lead to a sedentary lifestyle, other types, including mobile food journals and fitness apps, can help you make healthy choices. If you need motivation, support and advice, technology can be a helpful asset. Habits like distracted eating and excessive cellphone use can make the pounds add up quickly. If used correctly, mobile health apps can help you improve the quality of your life. When it comes to weight loss and nutrition, technology can help you:

- Analyze your current eating and fitness patterns.

- Identify weaknesses and bad habits.

- Help you eliminate unhealthy foods from your diet.

- Increase your awareness of your current lifestyle.

Research also shows that sharing your weight loss efforts with friends can help you reach your goals. Many weight loss and nutrition apps have a social sharing feature, allowing you to connect with your like-minded friends who can provide the support you need.

A Good Night's Sleep

Sleep is an often-neglected lifestyle factor that also plays an important role during weight loss. The recommended sleep duration for adults is seven to nine hours a night, but many people often sleep far less than this. Research has shown that sleeping less than the recommended amount is linked to having greater body fat and increased risk of obesity. It can also influence how easily you lose weight on a calorie-controlled diet. Typically, the goal for weight loss is to decrease body fat while retaining as much muscle mass as possible. Not getting the right amount of sleep can determine how much fat is lost as well as how much muscle mass you retain while on a calorie restricted diet (Chokroverty, 2006).

There are several reasons why fewer hours of sleep may be associated with higher body weight and may affect weight loss. These include changes in metabolism, appetite, and food selection.

Sleep influences two important appetite hormones in our body, leptin and ghrelin. Leptin is a hormone that decreases appetite, so when leptin levels are high we usually feel fuller. On the other hand, ghrelin is a hormone that can stimulate appetite, and is often referred to as the "hunger hormone" because it's thought to be responsible for the feeling of hunger.

One study (Chokroverty, 2006) found that sleep restriction increases levels of ghrelin and decreases leptin. Another study, which included a sample of 1,024 adults, also found that short sleep was associated with higher levels of ghrelin and lower levels of leptin. This combination could increase a person's appetite, making calorie-restriction more difficult to adhere to and may make a person more likely to overeat.

Consequently, increased food intake due to changes in appetite hormones may result in weight gain. This means that, in the long term, sleep deprivation may lead to weight gain due to changes in appetite. So, getting a good night's sleep should be prioritized (Chokroverty, 2006).

Along with changes in appetite hormones, inadequate sleep has also been shown to impact food selection and the way the brain perceives food. Researchers have found that the areas of the brain responsible for reward are more active in response to food after sleep loss (six nights of only four hours' sleep) when compared to people who had good sleep (six nights of nine hours' sleep).

This could possibly explain why sleep-deprived people snack more often and tend to choose carbohydrate-rich foods and sweet-tasting snacks, compared to those who get enough sleep.

Less Stress

Stress is such an incredibly powerful influence that even if you are doing everything right in terms of diet, nutrition and exercise, it can still crush your efforts to stay healthy. Prolonged periods of high stress can contribute significantly and directly to many conditions, ranging from reduced quality of life to deadly diseases such as cancer, heart disease, Alzheimer's disease, and many others.

Stress contributes to fatigue, bacterial and viral infections, inflammatory illness, blood-sugar problems, weight gain, intestinal distress, headaches, and many other disorders. Stress-related problems account for more than 75% of all visits to primary-care physicians and are responsible each day for millions of people needing to take time off work and school. So, stress comes with a monetary price tag as well as a toll on your health.

Charles Darwin said it's not the fittest who survive, nor the most intelligent, but those who can best adapt to their environment. Today, we refer to this adaptation as coping.

It's important to remember that stress is a normal part of life and health, and excess stress is not without remedy. The body has a great coping mechanism for stress—the hormones of the adrenal glands and related nervous system function. However, when the adrenal glands are overworked, bodywide problems can result.

Being more aware of your physical, chemical and mental stress is a big step for improving health. Reducing or eliminating individual stresses is easier if you write them down on paper. On a page, make three columns, one each for physical, chemical, and mental stresses. In each category, write down your stresses. This may take several days to complete since you probably won't think of all your different stresses right away. When you're done, prioritize by placing the biggest stress of each category on top. Then, work on reducing or eliminating one stress at a time. Or, if you can handle it, work on one stress from each category at a time. Reducing or eliminating unnecessary stress from your life will give your body a better chance to cope with other stresses you may not be able to change right now.

As you make your list, put a star by the stresses over which you have some control. This may include unhealthy eating habits like rushing or skipping your meals, drinking too much coffee, or not taking time to exercise.

Simply draw a line through those stresses that you can't control. If there's nothing you can do about them anyway, don't worry about them for now. Many people expend lots of energy on stresses they can't do anything about. This may include job stress or the weather, though in reality, almost any stress can be modified or eliminated—it's just a question of how far you're willing to go for optimal health. As time goes on, you may want to reconsider some of the items you've crossed off. You'll realize that changing jobs is a must or moving to a more compatible climate is necessary for your health.

Once you can "see" any stress listed on paper, it will be easier to manage. Start with your starred stresses first, because you have control over them—not that it's always easy to control them. Circle the three biggest stresses from the starred list and begin to work on them. You may be able to improve on some and totally eliminate others. Some will require habit changes. It's a big task, but one that will give you great benefits. When you've succeeded in eliminating or modifying each stress, cross it off your list and circle the three next most stressful ones, so you always have three stresses to work on.

In addition to your stress list, you're probably familiar with other strategies for dealing with stress, though you may not use them. Let's look at them:

- Learn to say "no" when asked to do something you really don't want to do. Ask yourself if you really want to do something before committing to it.

- Decide not to waste your time worrying about the past or the future. That's not to say you should ignore the past or not plan for the future. Live in the present.

- Learn some relaxation techniques and perform them regularly. The most powerful one is the respiratory biofeedback that we already discussed. A walk in nature can also be a great way to relax.

- When you're concerned about something, talk it over with someone you trust.

- Simplify your life. Start by eliminating trivia. Ask yourself: "Is this really important?"

- Prioritize your busy schedule; do the most important things first, but don't neglect the enjoyable things. Before getting out of bed in the morning, ask yourself: "What fun things do I have planned for today?"

- Know your passion and pursue it.

What's most important about stress is that too much of it interferes with rest. Or more accurately, recovering from excess stress requires more rest. If you don't get enough rest, usually in the form of sleep, the effects of stress will continue accumulating. One of the questions to ask yourself is whether you're getting enough sleep, considering the amount of stress you have. As you will see, one of the symptoms of excess stress is insomnia.

By learning to take control of the various types of stresses in your life, you can improve the quality of your life, reduce the risk of dysfunction and disease, and also help your adrenal glands regulate stress. Maintaining proper adrenal function is central to optimal fitness and health.

Implementation of these additional aids in your new lifestyle will solve one of your major life problems, obesity. You will also resolve many common signs and symptoms that reduce quality of life in general. Try to implement at least one of them by the end of this month. You will see the benefits and you will immediately want to add the others. The more you practice them and the sooner you act on them, the better.

CHAPTER SEVEN
Exercising and Weight Loss

I

t's clear that regular aerobic exercise is essential for you to attain optimal fitness and health. But I want to re-emphasize that I'm not talking about a no-pain, no-gain exercise program that will fall by the wayside as quickly as you start it. Instead, incorporate into your lifestyle an ongoing, long-term natural aerobic exercise routine that will greatly improve your energy levels, staminaand endurance, while helping you tone the aerobic muscles and train your body to burn more fat for energy. Physical activity should be something that you look forward to. It is the only way to embrace it for a lifetime.

Exercise programs are quite individual. Some people just want to stay fit and healthy and keep their weight in check. Others have goals such as training for the Ironman Triathlon. For either of these types, and for everyone in between, many basic principles are the same. All people who exercise want to gradually build up to a specific level, using the 180 Formula to improve aerobic fitness. Additionally, anyone on an exercise plan needs to balance this program with everything else in his or her life, including proper rest and recovery. I've trained many world class and professional athletes using the same principles outlined in this book; likewise for those just starting out. The volume of training is the difference. For serious athletes, training paces get significantly faster as their aerobic systems improve (Kelly A., Gennat, O'Rourke, Del Mar, 2006).

Finding Out Your Way to Exercise

Nothing is better than walking for overall fitness and health. Of all the types of exercise, walking is the one I recommend the most and not just for beginners, but for regular exercisers and even professional athletes. It's the most fail-safe exercise. Scientific studies show that walking burns a higher percentage of fat than any other activity because of its low intensity. Walking activates the small aerobic muscle fibers, which often are not stimulated by higher-intensity aerobic workouts. Walking also helps circulate blood, process lactic acid, and improve lymph drainage (important to the body's waste-removal system).

Walking is one of the best ways to get started on an exercise program since it's a simple, low-stress workout that is not easily overdone. Walkers generally have little difficulty keeping their heart rates from getting too high, though there are exceptions. The only problem with walking is that the heart rate won't go high enough into the maximum aerobic range (which isn't absolutely necessary). The mechanics of walking result in less gravity stress than you experience when jogging or running, but still enough to give you the important fat-burning benefits, as well as others, such as bone-strengthening effects.

We've all heard and read about the many wonderful benefits of exercise. But did you know most studies that demonstrate these great benefits were achieved through walking? You don't need to make exercise complicated, expensive, or intense. And I'm talking about just an easy walk—not power walking, race walking, or carrying weights. Here are some of the facts about the benefits of easy walking:

- **Regular, easy walking increases life expectancy.** It also helps older adults maintain their functional independence, an important concern for society. Currently, the average number of non-functional years in our elderly population is about 12. That's a dozen years at the end of a lifespan of doing nothing: unable to care for yourself, walk, be productive, or just enjoy life.

- **Regular, easy physical exercise such as walking can help prevent and manage coronary heart disease, the leading cause of death in the United States, as well as hypertension, diabetes, osteoporosis and depression.** This occurs through improved balance of blood fats, better clotting factors, improved circulation, and the ability to more efficiently regulate blood sugar.

- **Regular exercise like walking decreases your risk of developing degenerative disease.** The lack of exercise places more people at risk for coronary heart disease than all other risk factors. Aerobic deficiency is an independent risk for coronary heart disease, doubling the risk. Inactivity poses the same risk for coronary heart disease as smoking and hypertension.

- **Walking is associated with a lower rate of colon cancer, stroke, and low-back injury.**

All this can be accomplished with easy aerobic exercise. How easy? The equivalent of a sustained 30-minute walk, four or five times a week. Less than 30% of Americans are this active, including children who spend most of their spare time watching TV (Kelly A., Gennat, O'Rourke, Del Mar, 2006).

For some people, especially those who have been very inactive, very overweight, or chronically ill, even walking may pose overexertion problems. Whether 18 or 80, if you're beginning an exercise program, or have been inactive for a period of time and now want to start walking, consider using a heart monitor to take the guesswork out of your walk. I've seen too many beginners walking with a high heart rate. It's often because they're with other people and the instinct to be competitive comes into play. Talking while walking also increases the heart rate, and so does walking up a hill too fast before some level of fitness has been achieved. Former athletes seeking to restore their fitness can benefit from walking; it keeps them from being too aggressive early in their programs. The most important thing for a walker to realize is that it's a fat-burning and endurance routine. Don't worry about speed; instead, concern yourself with endurance. Base your walking on time rather than miles.

Balanced Exercise and Health

Working out adds many new dimensions to your life—an important component of optimal human performance. Much like diet and nutrition, each person must find an individualized program to meet his or her particular needs. So, start out as simply as possible. Then consider joining a group to get some psychological encouragement, as long as you can exercise within your own limits. Through this habit change, the exercise program becomes a positive addiction. Your routine will ultimately become a part of your day, like brushing your teeth.

There are a number of important factors to consider when starting or modifying your exercise routine:

- **Scheduling.** Create a realistic schedule of exercise that fits your family, work, and other commitments. This will allow you to be more consistent and help make it part of a new lifestyle.

- **Physical factors.** Be sure you can withstand the minor stress of exercise. Do you have some physical imbalances that may be aggravated by exercise? Take into consideration a history of prior injuries or conditions. Consider your workout surface—blacktop, wood, and carpet are preferable to concrete, marble, and steel. Grass and dirt surfaces may be safe, but they can also be stressful if they are uneven or too soft.

- **Chemical factors.** The proper nutrients, especially fats, are necessary for aerobic efficiency. High-sugar foods and drinks can be detrimental when consumed before workouts. Proper hydration is a must; drink water all day, not just after working out.

- **Psychological factors.** Studies have shown that people who exercise in the morning find it easier to maintain a regular program. But whether you exercise in the morning, midday or evening, be consistent. Write out a simple exercise program, if necessary. You are more apt to follow something you can see. Keep a log on a calendar or in a diary to see your success as the days, weeks, and months go by.

- **Goals.** Set realistic goals. Some people merely want to progress to exercising 30 minutes a day. Be conservative, but don't hesitate to dream. Running a marathon after six months of training may be realistic only for very disciplined people who can control their stress. You won't break any records and completing the marathon should be your only goal. I've worked with many patients who successfully met that goal in a healthy way.

- **Habit changes.** Starting an exercise program is, first of all, a change of habit. And as we all know, a habit change can be the most difficult change to make—even more difficult than the exercise itself. Generally, there are two barriers. One is just getting started and the other is when your enthusiasm wears off a bit. (Although being aware of this is usually incentive enough to keep going.)

- **Time.** Most exercise should be measured in time, and not miles, laps, or repetitions (except when performing your MAF Test). At the onset, a minimal time is best, since the purpose initially is to develop an exercise habit. The only exception may be if you progress to anaerobic workouts, such as weightlifting, where a range of measurements should always be used. This gives you more choice, allowing for daily fluctuations in energy level and time restraints. For example, when using weights, the number of repetitions may be 10 to 15, rather than doing a predetermined exact number based on some program not meant for you.

- **Intensity.** The intensity of your workout is an important consideration, as measured by the heart rate. Make sure you understand how to find your maximum aerobic heart rate using the 180 Formula. Base your exercise program on time and intensity (as per heart rate); e.g., 30 minutes of walking at a heart rate of under 140 beats per minute, five times per week.

A Beginner's World

Even if you've never been active, aerobic exercise is easy and simple. You can always take a walk. You can do this on your way to work, or on your way home, as part of your lunch break, or any time, really. It can be performed walking indoors or outdoors. You can also use a treadmill or stationary bike, either in your home or at the gym. A simple aerobic workout will easily fit into your current work schedule and requires no special equipment, clothing, or gear. Here is a typical starting program for a beginner:

- 30 minutes easy walking.
- 12-minute warm-up period, 12-minute cool-down period.
- Heart rate not to exceed the maximum aerobic level.
- A Monday through Friday schedule.
- Saturdays and Sundays off.

You can always fit in a 30-minute workout at some point during the day. Within that time, include at least a 12-minute warm-up period, where your activity level is very low. For the next 6 minutes move at a faster pace, but not so fast that it becomes uncomfortable—there's no need to break a sweat and you should be able to carry on a conversation. The remaining 12 minutes is your cool-down, another period of very low activity. This is an optimal aerobic workout—one that you can do in your work clothes during the course of the day.

Remember, your basic beginning program should be tailored to your specific needs. While most people are capable of at least 30 minutes of walking, perhaps 45 minutes is a good starting point. The maximum starting point for other beginners is an hour. Still others may benefit starting with 20 minutes per session. If you are recovering from a chronic illness or have been very inactive all your life, you should consider only 15 minutes of exercise, or even 10 minutes, as a start, and also consult your doctor

How rapidly you increase the time period depends on your response. Whatever the starting point, assuming that proper time is chosen, maintain that time for at least three weeks. Listen to your body; it will tell you if and when you can increase your exercise. This is also true for any change. Maintain the new time for at least three weeks before increasing it if there's no difficulty.

Don't increase the time you exercise by more than 50% at any one time in a program of up to 45 minutes, and not more than 15 minutes when the program is 45 minutes or more. Some people are quite content with 45 minutes. This is fine since you can obtain many benefits when exercising at this level five times per week.

What type of exercise should you do? When starting out, do almost anything, as long as it's aerobic. This may include, besides walking, riding a stationary bike, dancing, rebounding (trampoline), outdoor biking, swimming, hiking, cross-country skiing, and using various exercise machines. Jogging, or running, when done aerobically, is a healthy exercise. There is no universally accepted scientific distinction between running and jogging.

For the purposes of this book, I refer to jogging when I mean a much slower pace than running. Running occurs with progression and more speed and involves a slightly different gait. Any combination of these activities is also acceptable, as long as your heart rate doesn't exceed your maximum aerobic level. If you wish, do two or three types of exercise throughout the week or even in one workout. For example, you can walk for 15 minutes, ride a stationary bike for 20 minutes and dance for 15 minutes. This "cross-training" routine is actually healthier than doing just one exercise each session.

Anaerobic activities, including any type of weight-lifting, sit-ups, pushups, or activities that raise the heart rate above your maximum aerobic heart rate are not acceptable substitutes for aerobic exercise. They shouldn't be started until after you have developed your aerobic system. For the beginner, my recommendation is to wait at least six months and for those modifying their program, wait at least three to four months before performing any anaerobic work.

Tennis, racquetball, and similar sports often end up being anaerobic for the beginner, because of the type of muscle fibers used and the high heart rates produced. They're fun to do, but should be considered "games" and not exercise unless they're performed regularly; e.g., if you walk four times per week, play tennis once a week, or do 18 holes of golf once a week. In that case, a proper warm-up and cooldown is important and so are regulating aerobic and anaerobic levels. Once you have progressed through a certain number of weeks without any problems, you may want to further develop your health and fitness.

Final Words

T he more weight you gain, the more dangerous it becomes. Extra weight spells illness, whether it is in the form of diabetes or a heart condition. They will happen if you don't do something about it. To lose weight, you have to be proactive. This is not necessarily about being toned and sculpted, but about maintaining a weight that is not life-threatening. You can work on the abs later, right now you just need to shed some body fat.

When it comes to weight loss programs, I have a lot of things to say. Weight loss programs must focus on helping women achieve energy balance as well as weight loss and mental health. But in order to do achieve this balance, a number of approaches can be used. Often, these approaches do not work and women fail to lose weight. In this chapter, I will explain the process of weight loss, calorie counting, and how I manage my weight.

In fact, my program is a simple weight loss program powered by the benefits of non-dairy keto recipes. This weight loss program will give you information on your dietary intake to help you on your weight loss journey.

The Process of Losing Weight

About 70% of the calories you burn each day go toward merely keeping you alive. This is called the basal metabolic rate (BMR). These are things like breathing, circulation, and maintaining body temperature (generating heat). It also allows you to produce new cells and recycle old ones; adjust hormone levels, brain, and nerve function; and sedentary tasks like sleeping, sitting, or checking your smartphone.

About 20% of calories are consumed for physical actions, like walking to the train, doing chores, or exercising. This is the factor you can control with increased activity. But unless you spend the entire day in the gym, it will never rival the calorie consumption of simply existing.

And finally, about 10% of calories are used for digesting your food. This doesn't vary much, whether you are eating "negative calorie foods," like celery that are said to take more calories to digest than they supply, or cupcakes. But that doesn't mean you should binge on cupcakes. Understanding the actual process of losing weight is important to begin with the actual weight loss process as it will help you design a regimen that works best for you. Yes, I am talking about exercises and recipes.

When we think about weight loss, the assumption is that we'll be losing fat. However, it is much more complicated than that since not all weight loss is necessarily fat loss. In an ideal world, the body would only burn fat, we'd lose belly fat, and it would be easy to look fit. Unfortunately, that's not the case. Your weight is determined by the rate at which you store energy from the food you eat and the rate at which you use this energy for your body functioning. Remember that when your body breaks down fat, each fat cell gets smaller, but the number of fat cells still remains the same (Wing, O.Hill, 2001).

When we eat sugars and starches, our body breaks them into glucose, which is the easiest fuel for our cells tooxidize for energy. Now, if we eat too many calories, our bodies convert the excess glucose into fatty acids and lock them away as adipose tissue for later. Excess amino acids from protein can also be converted into fatty acids.

As long as we have excess energy, regardless of its form, fat cells keep growing. This process of handling excess carbohydrates in the blood and the inhibition of the breakdown of fat is controlled by a hormone signaling system, which includes insulin as one of the primary signals. After a meal, the elevated blood sugar triggers insulin release, which tells the fat cells to hold onto their energy stores and the muscle and other tissues to absorb and burn the glucose first.

Once the level of glucose in the blood drops, insulin levels drop as well and then the body starts to mobilize energy from your fat cells. This is a complex process triggered by a number of hormones and carried out by enzymes and coenzymes, first by unlocking the fat cells, transporting fatty acids into cells, and finally breaking them down into smaller units for consumption. Remember that fat cells will not release their energy stores if insulin is present. So, a diet that can keep your blood sugar stable is the key to fat loss. This means that you need to avoid sugar, refined carbs, and other fast-digesting packaged foods (Wing, O.Hill, 2001).

When you get started on a diet plan and reduce your calories, the body can burn fat, but it can also burn muscle tissue if you starve yourself. This is a cruel trick of nature and one of the major reasons why crash dieters tend to regain their weight. Losing muscle mass can lead to a slow metabolic rate. When you are not eating properly or you are crash-dieting, your body is not absorbing food. When this happens, the insulin amount in the bloodstream is very low and the energy required for body functioning is consumed from internal stores of complex carbs, fats, and proteins. Under these conditions, some organs of your body secrete hormones:

- Pancreas: glucagon
- Pituitary gland: growth hormone
- Pituitary gland: ACTH (adrenocorticotropic hormone)
- Adrenal gland: epinephrine (adrenaline)
- Thyroid gland: thyroid hormone

These hormones act on cells in the liver, muscle and fat tissue, and have the opposite effects of insulin (Wing, O.Hill, 2001).

So, you should be suspicious of any fad diet promising extreme weight loss in a very short time period, as it is not a sustainable solution and is likely stealing from your future for the illusion of results in the present. To lose weight safely and sustain that weight loss over time, it is important to make some gradual, permanent, and beneficial changes to your lifestyle.

Another reason the scale might show a lower value is loss of water. Water molecules are both bound up in fat and glucose, as well as attached to them. Whenever we burn these fuels, carbon and water are released. We breathe out the carbon as CO_2 and eliminate the water through urine and sweat. When you first start a diet, weight loss appears to be more rapid in the first two weeks because the extra water that's been bound up in your body is being released as your energy stores are tapped. This is a good and perfectly natural thing. This is also why you may find your weight jump up again if you have a cheat day or binge at a birthday party. Water molecules will attach to any new fat or glycogen you store, raising the number on the scale faster than you might expect after a binge.

Weight gain and weight loss are complicated. The process is controlled by food composition, hormone signaling, calorie balance, and your lifestyle, which includes sleep, physical activity and stress. There's nothing wrong with slow weight loss, other than feelings of despair that could accompany lack of progress. In fact, slow weight loss helps to keep your metabolism high. But with science on our side, we can maximize the rate of healthy, responsible fat loss to get you to your goal weight both quickly and safely. This will set you up for a lifetime of healthy weight maintenance, with no rebound or weight regain. If you examine the most responsible diet plans, you will find good food as the foundation.

Calorie Counting: Why is it important?

Body weight is primarily determined by a simple concept known as energy balance. Energy balance is the ratioof energy ingested through foods and beverages to the energy expended through basal metabolism, the thermic effect of food, and physical activity.

The energy discussed in nutrition and weight management is measured in kilocalories (kcal). One kcal is defined as the amount of heat, or energy, necessary to raise 1 kg of water by 1°C. Although the scientifically correct term for this energy is kcal, most consumer-facing and educational resources refer to this as simply calories. For this reason, nutrition facts labels will display energy in terms of calories per serving and calories from fat, as opposed to using kcal (Bray, G. 1969).

Energy Ingested

Energy or calories ingested by human beings come from four macronutrients: carbohydrate, fat, protein, and alcohol. Based on its corresponding chemical structure, each of these macronutrients will provide a particular level of energy or calories per gram ingested.

Carbohydrates and protein are the least energy-dense of the macronutrients, providing ~4 kcal/g. Alcohol provides 7 kcal/g. Fat is the most energy-dense providing ~9 kcal/g.

The caloric content of foods and beverages is based on the grams of carbohydrate, fat, protein, and alcohol in the associated product.

For example, if a food's nutrition facts label states that it has 25 g of carbohydrate (CHO), 1 g of fat (FAT), 1 g of protein (PRO), and no alcohol per single serving, then one serving of that food should have 113 kcal (although, due to the rounding of some of these numbers, the label may state that the caloric content is slightly higher or lower than this number).

Carbohydrates

Carbohydrates and carbohydrate-containing foods are extremely important to the American diet. In general, most Americans consume plenty of carbohydrates each day; however, the types of carbohydrate-containing foods Americans typically eat are not considered ideal. As such, when discussing weight management and obesity prevention, it is imperative to discuss carbohydrates and carbohydrate-containing foods in order to better understand what dietary modifications should be made (Bray, G. 1969).

Chemically speaking, carbohydrates are made up of single or strands of carbon rings, called saccharide polymers. These polymers take on four different forms: a single saccharide polymer (monosaccharides), two polymers attached to each other (disaccharides), three to nine polymers in a single strand (oligosaccharides), or ten or more polymers in a single strand (polysaccharides).

Monosaccharide and disaccharide polymers are commonly referred to as simple carbohydrates or simple sugars. Monosaccharide polymers include the most elemental forms of carbohydrate found in nature: glucose, galactose, and fructose. Disaccharide polymers are made up of two monosaccharide polymers joined together, and the three disaccharides are sucrose (glucose + fructose), lactose (glucose + galactose), and maltose (glucose + glucose).

On the nutrition facts label, the monosaccharide and disaccharide content of a food will be indicated on the rows labeled "Total Sugars." It is important to note that total sugars include both the naturally occurring simple sugars (e.g., lactose in milk) and added sugars that are incorporated during food processing (e.g., high fructose corn syrup in ketchup). Future labeling regulations may require manufacturers to distinguish between natural and added sugars, but as of the writing of this book, the current nutrition facts label combines these two sugars. Oligosaccharide and polysaccharide polymers contain three or more monosaccharide units; thus they are referred to as complex carbohydrates (Bray, G. 1969).

Oligosaccharides, which contain three to nine monosaccharide polymers, are commonly found in legumes. Polysaccharides, the longest chains of saccharide polymers, are often called starch and are commonly found in starchy vegetables (e.g., potatoes and peas) and grains (e.g., breads, pasta, and rice).

Fats

Dietary fats are an essential component of any healthy diet. Although dietary fat gained a negative connotation in the 1990s and early 2000s, researchers have shown fat to be a key element in weight management. Fat is known as one of the dietary components that leads to satiety, or feelings of fullness after a meal (Bray, G. 1969). Fat also contributes to food's palatability and desirable texture. Nonetheless, when talking about fat, you should realize that not all fats are created equal. Some fats appear to have more health consequences than others. As such, you should be careful and primarily focus on consuming healthy fats.

Dietary fats basically fall into three main categories: unsaturated, saturated, and trans. Unsaturated fats are made up of carbon chains containing at least one double bond. Monounsaturated fats contain just one double bond, while polyunsaturated fats contain multiple double bonds. Saturated fats do not contain any double bonds and are simply long chains of carbon linked solely by single bonds. Trans fats are similar to unsaturated fats in that they do contain at least one double bond; however, they also undergo a configuration change during processing.

It is important to recognize that foods are typically made up of a combination of fats and rarely contain one single type of fat. For example, olive oil is commonly referred to as a good source of monounsaturated fat; however, it also contains a small amount of saturated fat. Similarly, lard is commonly referred to as a source of saturated fat, but it also contains some monounsaturated fats and polyunsaturated fats (Bray, G. 1969).

Not all dietary fats are created equal, and some are known to contribute to more health problems than others. For example, the 2010 Dietary Guidelines for Americans recommend that individuals limit their saturated fat intake to no more than 10% of their calories because saturated fat has been associated with poor health outcomes (Dietary Guidelines for Americans, 2010), including cardiovascular disease and stroke. The Guidelines also recommend Americans limit their trans-fat intake as much as possible because of similar poor health associations. Because saturated and trans-fat intake should be limited, Americans should replace them with monounsaturated and polyunsaturated fats. Sources of these fats tend to have a higher nutritional value and are not associated with the same health consequences.

Among the polyunsaturated fats, omega 3 and omega 6 fatty acids are known as the essential fats. These two fatty acids cannot be synthesized by the body yet are essential to health. As such, these two polyunsaturated fats must be consumed through the diet. Alpha-linolenic acid (ALA), eicosatetraenoic acid (EPA), and docosahexaenoic acid (DHA) are three of the omega 3 fatty acids, and these omega 3s can be found in fish (e.g., salmon) as well as plant oils (e.g., flaxseed oil). Omega 3 fatty acids have received a lot of attention due to their associations with improving fetal development and reducing inflammation and, as a result, are commonly sold in supplement form. Unlike omega 3 fatty acids, most Americans consume sufficient amounts of omega 6 fatty acids. Linolenic acid, one of the most commonly consumed omega 6 fatty acids, is readily found in meat and dairy products (Bray, G. 1969).

Proteins

Protein, the third essential macronutrient, is essential for building new body tissue. Similar to the proteins found in the body, dietary proteins are made up of long chains of amino acids, also called polypeptides. There are 20 amino acids that make up these polypeptides. While all amino acids are structurally similar, the differentiating characteristic is each amino acid's unique side group.

Amino acids fall intoone of three categories: essential, nonessential, and conditionally essential. Essential amino acids are ones that cannot be synthesized in the human body, and therefore, must be ingested through the diet. There are nine essential amino acids. Nonessential amino acids are ones that the body can make in sufficient amounts to meet human needs and, therefore, do not have to be ingested. Conditionally essential amino acids are similar to nonessential amino acids in that they are typically produced in sufficient amounts by the human body; however, under stressful situations, the body may not be able to produce sufficient amounts. Thus, in order to meet the body's demands in times of stress, individuals should consume these amino acids through the diet (Bray, G. 1969).

Now, let's talk about counting calories. Yes, you should definitely do it! Why? Counting calories is necessary because it ensures you're eating the amount you think you're eating. A common problem is incorrectly estimating or guessing calorie intake. Dieters typically underestimate the amount they're eating because they assume it's impossible for foods to have as many calories as they actually do.

For example, pizza contains about 400 calories per slice. A 1/4 cup of peanuts contains almost 200 calories. A footlong sub contains around 1,000 calories. It's very common for some foods to provide a third or even half of your daily calorie allotment. Ignoring, underestimating or guessing calorie intake leads to slow or non-existent weight loss. An important part of weight balance is looking at the nutrition label, figuring out how much one serving actually is (with the help of measuring cups, spoons, and food scales) and counting calories to ensure you're eating the proper amount. If weight control isn't going as planned, the likely culprit is eating an inappropriate number of calories. Counting calories isn't as tedious as it once used to be. There are plenty of apps for this purpose, making calorie counting much easier today than in the past.

Overtime, your ability to estimate calorie intake improves. At the beginning of your weight management journey (gaining, losing, or maintaining weight), it's important to avoid estimating intake and instead, carefully track calories and food. However, do not overdo this to the point where you don't even want to sit down to eat because the process of tracking everything is exhausting to you. Moderation applies here just as much as it does everywhere else.

In conclusion, there are a multitude of reasons why we should change our diet to a healthier one, but the number one reason for all of us should be as simple as the fact that we want a great quality of life as we age. We all may have seen people running back and forth to hospital for cancer treatments and other illnesses or heard about people getting body parts amputated because of diabetes. We also know people who take a handful of drugs every day to stay alive. Ask yourself this: do you see yourself depending on medications to be alive? Do you want to be that person that has to inject themselves with insulin? Most of us don't want to think about these things, but these are the things that come from eating the wrong stuff.

If you are serious about turning your life around, take it slowly. Try eliminating two items each week until you have eliminated all of the flour, milk, pasta, sugar, and rice products. Ask a friend to join you for support or just root for yourself. Many of us fail before we ever give it a good try, so from a woman to another woman, just try it. You deserve a healthy body and a happy life and they are within your reach if you follow the advice laid out in this book. Staying fit and happy after 40 as a woman is a great decision to make and will ensure that you have decades of healthy living in front of you. You deserve it! Now that you have the tools, go out and use them. If you enjoyed this book, please leave a review on Amazon.

Reference List

Redman L, Heilbronn L, Martin C, et al. . Effects of calorie restriction with or without exercise on body composition and fat distribution. J Clin Endorcrinol Metab 2007;92:865–872

Newsholme, Eric Arthur, and Carole Start. Regulation in metabolism. 1973.

Smith, Reuben L; Soeters, Maarten R; Wüst, Rob C I; Houtkooper, Riekelt H (24 April 2018). "Metabolic flexibility as an adaptation to energy resources and requirements in health and disease". Endocrine Reviews. 39 (4): 489–517. doi:10.1210/er.2017-00211

Mozaffarian, Dariush, Tao Hao, Eric B. Rimm, Walter C. Willett, and Frank B. Hu. "Changes in diet and lifestyle and long-term weight gain in women and men." New England Journal of Medicine 364, no. 25 (2011): 2392-2404.

Jeffery RW, Adlis SA, Forster JL. Prevalence of dieting among working men and women: The Healthy Worker Project. Health Psychol.

1991;10:274–281. doi: 10.1037/0278-6133.10.4.274.

NHLBI. 2013. Managing Overweight and Obesity in Adults: Systematic Evidence Review from the Obesity Expert Panel.

Gao, Dengfeng, Ning Ning, Congxia Wang, Yuhuan Wang, Qing Li, Zhe Meng, Yang Liu, and Qiang Li. "Dairy products consumption and risk of type 2 diabetes: systematic review and dose-response meta-analysis." PloS one 8, no. 9 (2013): e73965.

Kissebah, Ahmed H., David S. Freedman, and Alan N. Peiris. "Health risks of obesity." Medical Clinics of North America 73, no. 1 (1989): 111-138.

Shaw, Kelly A., Hanni C. Gennat, Peter O'Rourke, and Chris Del Mar. "Exercise for overweight or obesity." Cochrane database of systematic reviews 4 (2006).

Maughan, Ron J., Doug S. King, and Trevor Lea. "Dietary supplements." Journal of sports sciences 22, no. 1 (2004): 95-113.

Chokroverty, Sudhansu. "Overview of sleep & sleep disorders." Indian J Med Res 131, no. 2 (2010): 126-140.

Deikman, Arthur J. "Experimental meditation." Journal of Nervous and Mental Disease (1963).

German, J. Bruce, and Rosemary L. Walzem. "The health benefits of wine." Annual review of nutrition 20, no. 1 (2000): 561-593.

"History of the Ketogenic Diet" Epilepsia, Volume49, Issues8

Wing, Rena R., and James O. Hill. "Successful weight loss maintenance." Annual review of nutrition 21, no. 1 (2001): 323-341.

Bray, G. 1969. "Effect of Caloric Restriction on Energy Expenditure in Obese Patients." The Lancet 294, no. 7617, pp. 397–98. doi:10.1016/s0140-6736(69)90109-3

Freeman, John M., Eric H. Kossoff, and Adam L. Hartman. "The ketogenic diet: one decade later." Pediatrics 119, no. 3 (2007): 535-543.